Benjamin Waterhouse and the Introduction of Vaccination

YALE UNIVERSITY DEPARTMENT OF THE HISTORY OF MEDICINE MONOGRAPH SERIES NO. 33

Benjamin Waterhouse and the Introduction of Vaccination

A Reappraisal

by

JOHN B. BLAKE

PHILADELPHIA
UNIVERSITY OF PENNSYLVANIA PRESS

Published in Great Britain, India, and Pakistan
by the Oxford University Press
London, Bombay, and Karachi

Library of Congress Catalogue Card Number 57-7460

Printed in the United States of America
American Book–Stratford Press, Inc., New York

Acknowledgments

One of the historian's most pleasant duties is acknowledging the help he has received from others. Particularly does this apply to the libraries and their staffs who have made his research possible. The Massachusetts Historical Society, the Harvard Medical School Library, the Boston Public Library, the Boston Medical Library, the Library of the New York Academy of Medicine, and the Rhode Island Historical Society have all generously allowed me to use manuscripts in their possession. To the Sterling Memorial Library at Yale I am indebted particularly for the use of the newspaper collection, and especially must I thank Miss Madeline E. Stanton and Mrs. Henrietta T. Perkins of the Yale Medical Library, and Miss Elizabeth H. Thomson of the Department of the History of Medicine at Yale, for their unfailing courtesy and attention to many requests. Throughout this project, Dr. John F. Fulton has given me his enthusiastic encouragement and steady support.

While working on this study, I have been aided by a James Hudson Brown Memorial Research Fellowship from the Yale University School of Medicine, and by a fellowship from the Commonwealth Fund.

Plates

Benjamin Waterhouse
and the
Introduction of Vaccination

I

IN JULY, 1800, DR. BENJAMIN WATERHOUSE, HARVARD'S first Professor of the Theory and Practice of Physic, introduced the practice of vaccination against smallpox into the United States. Innumerable articles, pamphlets, and books have recorded this fact, and few events in American medical history are more commonly known.[1] As early as 1817 T. J. Pettigrew noted in his memoir of John C. Lettsom that the vaccine lymph spread from Waterhouse "through the United States." [2] Waterhouse received full credit in John Baron's life of Edward Jenner,[3] and more recent British writers have afforded him similar recognition.[4]

For many years, however, American authors granted Waterhouse little more than passing notice. Although Josiah Bartlett of Charlestown, Massachusetts, mentioned him generously in 1810,[5] and James Thacher named him as the nation's first vaccinator,[6] the *Boston Medical and Surgical Journal*, while recalling his "early and decided" advocacy of vaccination and his designation as the "American Jenner," gave him only a brief obituary.[7] Oliver Wendell Holmes in 1869 at least referred to Waterhouse's achievement,[8] but he received remarkably scant and slighting treatment in Edward Warren's biographies of his distinguished father and brother.[9] Samuel D. Gross omitted Waterhouse from his selection of outstanding medical figures,[10] and the centennial history of American medicine mentioned him but once.[11]

Not until 1881 did Henry A. Martin present the first

extended notice of Waterhouse's work. After castigating the hereditary "Boston Clique" for its treatment of his hero, Martin recounted the vaccinator's struggles primarily in his own words, and reproduced several letters from Thomas Jefferson to document the story of their cooperation.[12] The same year, however, in an address to the Massachusetts Medical Society, Samuel Abbott Green also recognized Waterhouse's contribution and cited his books on vaccination.[13] Three years later Joseph Jones reprinted part of Martin's article and added new material on other early vaccinators.[14] Following their lead, William M. Welch published in 1885 a more complete account of Waterhouse's achievement and firmly entrenched his name in the annals of American medical history.[15] Since then innumerable authors have swelled the volume of praise, so that today Waterhouse is one of our leading medical heroes: a recent list of the twenty-five outstanding pioneers of public health in America, the consensus of a number of experts in the field, accords sixteenth place to the man who introduced vaccination.[16]

With few exceptions historians have portrayed Waterhouse as struggling against public and professional prejudice and hostility in Boston, in marked contrast to the friendship and support of Jefferson and Jenner. To account for this opposition writers have mentioned Waterhouse's adherence to the Society of Friends, his political support of the Jeffersonian Republicans, and petty personal jealousy aroused by his superior scientific qualifications, his skill in controversy, his appointment as a young Rhode Islander to the first Professorship of Physic at Harvard, and his recognition as "The American Jenner." Almost nowhere has it been intimated that any of his actions in connection with the introduction of vaccination offered the Bostonians any legitimate reasons, other than personal ones, for disliking or distrusting him.[17]

Accounts of Waterhouse's work, however, when not derived from purely secondary material, nearly always depend directly and almost exclusively on his own forceful version, on letters published by Baron and Pettigrew, and in a few instances on some of the manuscripts preserved by his family. Some years ago James A. Spalding [18] and Morris C. Leikind [19] published certain correspondence that calls for a reappraisal of the relations between Waterhouse and his professional brethren. This material, and much more in the files of Boston newspapers, has never been adequately analyzed.[20]

II

Early in 1799 Benjamin Waterhouse received a copy of Edward Jenner's *Inquiry into the Causes and Effects of the Variolæ Vaccinæ* from his London friend and correspondent, Dr. John C. Lettsom, and soon thereafter drew up a brief account of the new discovery, which the *Columbian Centinel*, a Boston newspaper, published on March 16, 1799.[21] Other reports soon followed, and by 1800 several American physicians were attempting to import cowpox virus. On July 8, 1800, Waterhouse achieved the first significant result when he vaccinated his son Daniel.[22] On August 2, after treating six more members of his household, he requested Dr. William Aspinwall, who maintained a hospital for this purpose in Brookline, to inoculate one of them with smallpox. The test was an unqualified success.[23]

As the news spread, practitioners soon deluged Waterhouse with requests for information and vaccine, but he was as yet unwilling to comply. Since, he explained, he had

> taken much pains in this business, run no small risk of reputation, as well as of personal feelings, there are few he trusts that will wonder he is anxious to have the matter under his own eye until the practice is more firmly established by the public opinion. A few unsuccessful cases at the beginning, deprived *Scotland* of the blessings of inoculation for the small-pox for more than 20 years.[24]

Many physicians nevertheless continued to apply. Among them was Lyman Spalding of Portsmouth, New

Hampshire, who first wrote Waterhouse on August 25 of his plan to operate a smallpox inoculation hospital in conjunction with a Dr. Cutter, and of his interest in vaccination. Soon after, he sent another letter asking for cowpox "matter," and on September 6 Waterhouse replied:

> I have only time to say that I have received your second letter, and that I will accomodate you with the matter &c at the same lay which has been offered to me but I declined, namely for *one quarter of the profits arising from* the inoculation & the contract to remain for 14 months from this time. Abandon the idea of inoculating for small-pox & throw all your attention to the Kine-pox.[25] If this idea suits you & Dr Cutter you shall be accomodated at once, for half a dozen practitioners stand ready to jump at that offer and two of them are not at very great distance from you.
>
> I haste I am yours &c
>
> Benjn. Waterhouse [26]

Four days later, dropping the idea of a partnership with Cutter, Spalding accepted these terms, but added, "on your part it is expected, that the like priviledge will not be granted to others in my vicinity." [27] This did not satisfy Waterhouse. He wanted young Spalding to join forces with an older and better established practitioner, who would bring in more business and therefore increase his share. After several more letters had passed between them, however, Waterhouse acceded to Spalding's insistence on a local monopoly and on September 25 sent him the virus in return for his written bond to pay one quarter of the profits.[28]

Meanwhile, Waterhouse allotted the rest of Strafford, Grafton, and Rockingham counties in New Hampshire, except for Hanover and its vicinity, to three brothers, Drs. Levi, Josiah, and Ezra Bartlett, and in exchange for similar bonds provided them with vaccine. Later, it appears, Dr.

Thomas Banning joined them. Other favored physicians included a Dr. Rowe in Vermont; and in Massachusetts, Stowe Ranney of Brentwood, Benjamin Billings of Mansfield, Ebenezer Perry of New Bedford, James Mann of Wrentham, and Zacheus Bartlett of Plymouth. Similar arrangements were presumably concluded with Dr. David King of Newport, Rhode Island, and a Dr. Dyer of Providence, while at least one small-town practitioner, less likely to attain an extensive practice, received the lymph for a flat fee of one hundred and fifty dollars. Nor were these cases exceptional. To Zacheus Bartlett, Waterhouse outlined his "custom of supplying practitioners" on October 1:

> I would just observe to you that I have made a contract with several practitioners in different states & counties, and most of them have agreed to give me *one quarter* of the *neat* profits, others have given me a specific sum. In none have I *less* than a quarter of the profits.[29]

While thus distributing vaccine to selected country physicians who were unable to compete with him, Waterhouse denied it to those in the capital. In these circumstances his Harvard colleague John Warren on August 20 wrote to his son, a medical student in London:

> The Cow or Kine pox is making some noise here. I wish you had thought of procuring and sending me some matter, as Dr Waterhouse is the only Physician who has received it from London and has begun to practice, and the other Physicians cannot readily obtain it. I should like to know from you what its present character is and if you can easily obtain it and send it in a closely sealed Phial. I may possibly have it in that way sooner than any other.[30]

At the same time another Boston physician, Samuel Brown, to whom the Humane Society of Massachusetts

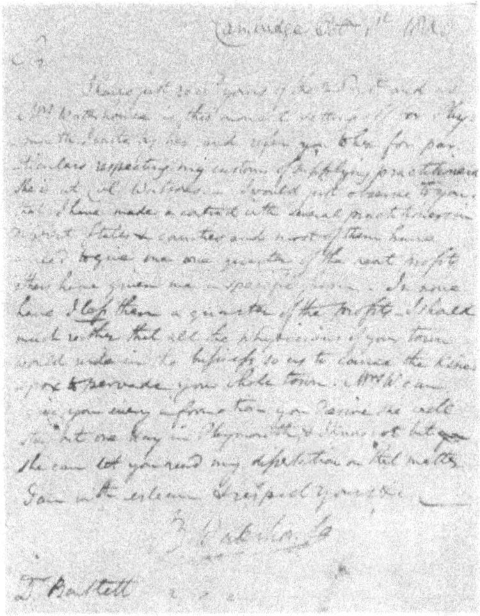

Plate I. Letter from Benjamin Waterhouse to Zacheus Bartlett, October 1, 1800. (Courtesy of New York Academy of Medicine.)

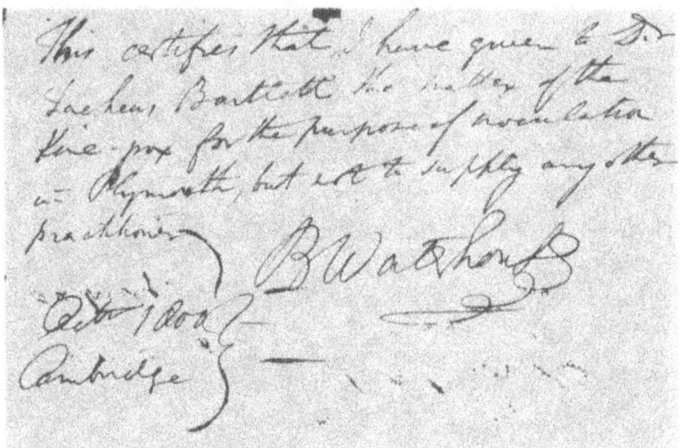

This certifies that I have given to Dr
Zacheus Bartlett the matter of the
kine-pox for the purpose of inoculation
in Plymouth, but not to supply any other
practitioner
B Waterhouse
Octr 1800
Cambridge

Plate II. Bartlett's certificate from Waterhouse, October, 1800. *(Courtesy of Dr. William Finkelstein.)*

had just awarded a prize for his treatise on yellow fever,[31] foiled in his attempt to obtain vaccine directly from the arms of some of Waterhouse's patients, advertised that if anyone having cowpox, "and not restricted to the contrary by oath, or solemn promise," would supply him with the "specific matter," he would "inoculate therewith *gratis*." Other physicians, he added, "without exception," might freely share in the vaccine thus produced.[32]

For this attempt to diffuse more widely the benefits of vaccination, an anonymous "Pedro" accused Brown of insolence, hypocrisy, arrogance, and quackery.

> The public too well know [the writer continued], to require further proof, with what industry and fortitude Dr. WATERHOUSE, in opposition to the most powerful prejudice, has reduced to a certainty the efficacious qualities of the matter produced from the *Kine Pox*. . . . And what animal could have been supposed sufficiently base, to wish to deprive the discoverer, or maturer of the discovery of a competent reward! . . . With the learned and captivating motto "PRO BONO PUBLICO," a stripling in his profession . . . offers, in terms of salvation, to heal the sick, assist the poor and needy, and even instruct his fathers and brethren of the lance, all *for nothing*, provided he can steal . . . something, that he never saw and knows nothing about! [33]

Apparently expecting this denunciation to have a salutary effect, Waterhouse noted in a letter to Lyman Spalding written the day it appeared that "Sam B.—— is in a fair way of being hooted out of Boston." But it did not entirely remove his apprehension. On September 12, insisting that Spalding's agreement to hand over the required percentage only until vaccination became public was "too vague," Waterhouse added, "Sam Brown may steal it before a month expires, and then in six months it may be diffused over Boston, or it may not." [34]

Soon it became evident, moreover, that others also endangered the monopoly. Having inaugurated the practice in Ipswich with vaccine direct from London, Dr. Thomas Manning advertised this fact in the *Columbian Centinel* on September 24. Still Waterhouse was not disheartened, since, as he wrote Spalding the next day, "Young Doctor Manning has the matter and will be as close with it as any of you, by what he says to me by letter." [35]

Hardly had Waterhouse penned this hopeful statement, when James Jackson returned from London. While there he had studied the new inoculation with Dr. William Woodville, one of its earliest and most important promoters, and, as he later wrote, "learned all then known about that business." Unfortunately Jackson's friends in Boston, though anxiously awaiting his return with vaccine, did not advise him of the local situation, and he brought only "a small piece of thread and four lancets charged with the matter." Arriving home on September 30, he discovered that "vaccination had just been introduced here, and Boston was full of it—so far as talking went." The next day he commenced practice.[36]

On October 7 Jackson hastily called upon his friend John Pickering in London to send more vaccine as soon as possible. "Everybody here," he wrote, "is in a rage to have the cow-pox. I brought matter here which has nearly failed and I fear will quite. If so, I may not be able to get a supply till this reaches me from London." [37] Learning the next day that his lymph had indeed failed, Jackson asked Waterhouse for a supply. The Cambridge professor apparently put him off with a promise, but his real attitude may be inferred from the triumphant note in his letter to Spalding of October 12: "Dr. Jackson *has not the matter*. He applied to me for it last week. He brought some, but it failed." [38]

Waterhouse was in part mistaken. As Jackson described it a month later,

Dr. Waterhouse had promised a supply, but I could not depend upon having it in season. I knew that Dr. Manning of Ipswich had received matter from his brother whom we saw in London; but it was said that he kept it to himself. Driven by despair, I went secretly to Ipswich determined to pay any price for a supply. My success was here as complete as unexpected. The Doctor gave all I asked and refused all compensation.[39]

Following this coup, Jackson on October 11 informed the public that he was prepared to inoculate for the cowpox.[40]

On the same day Warren informed his son that Jackson had begun to vaccinate. "Doctor Waterhouse," he wrote, "has made something handsome by it, (which he much needed) and it will probably be soon generally adopted here. He Dr Jackson . . . brought the *matter* with him—this has been hitherto monopolized but it will soon cease to be the case and there will be enough to be had by all the Physicians."[41] Warren's prediction proved true. Within a week other practitioners advertised their readiness to vaccinate, and by the middle of November Jackson noted that "the matter is now in the hands of all the physicians here."[42]

Throughout New England the monopoly was breaking down. From Stratham, New Hampshire, Josiah Bartlett in evident distress wrote to Spalding on November 3 that in his neighborhood many physicians were inoculating cowpox. They had, he thought, procured the virus in a "clandestine manner," and he added, "I believe that Doctor Manning has spread the Matter in this State, by way of Newbury. If he received the Matter from Dr. Waterhouse, as I heard that he did, and has spread it (as is reported of him) openly, Dr. Waterhouse ought to be informed of it."

Sorrowfully, Spalding replied that he too faced competition, "but in what manner Cutter or Dwight procured their infection, I cannot discover . . ." In these circumstances Josiah Bartlett concluded that it would be advisable to obtain Waterhouse's permission to sell the vaccine to other physicians. His brother Levi, believing this the only profitable recourse, concurred. Even then, he remarked, it soon would "not be so lucrative as other practice." According to the newspapers, he explained, "matter is dayly carried from Boston & disbursed to anyone who chuses. Dr. Hunt has been inoculating for the Kine Pox in Boston about three weeks without discrimination, Bond or any other security & anyone can I believe take matter from him. . . ." [43]

Though slow to accede to the Bartletts' request for permission to sell vaccine,[44] Waterhouse was apparently willing to have Spalding distribute it provided the recipients agreed to the usual terms. On October 25 one of Spalding's former students, Abraham Hedge of Chester, Vermont, had written to inquire how he could obtain the virus, "as it might now be of great service to me, and could not injure him [Waterhouse] or you, being at such a distance. It will soon doubtless become general," he pointed out, "when it can be no object." [45] On November 10 Spalding dispatched some virus to Hedge, and on the eighteenth the latter replied. He thanked Spalding for his description of cowpox and reported that he was seeking the town's permission to test some of his patients by variolation to convince the local people of the efficacy of vaccination. But he added, "The price you or your friends set on the infection sent me would have been gladly paid, had not I already received a supply which, that you may not think I act the rogue, I will inform you where I got it." His sources were Dr. Nathan Smith of Hanover (who ob-

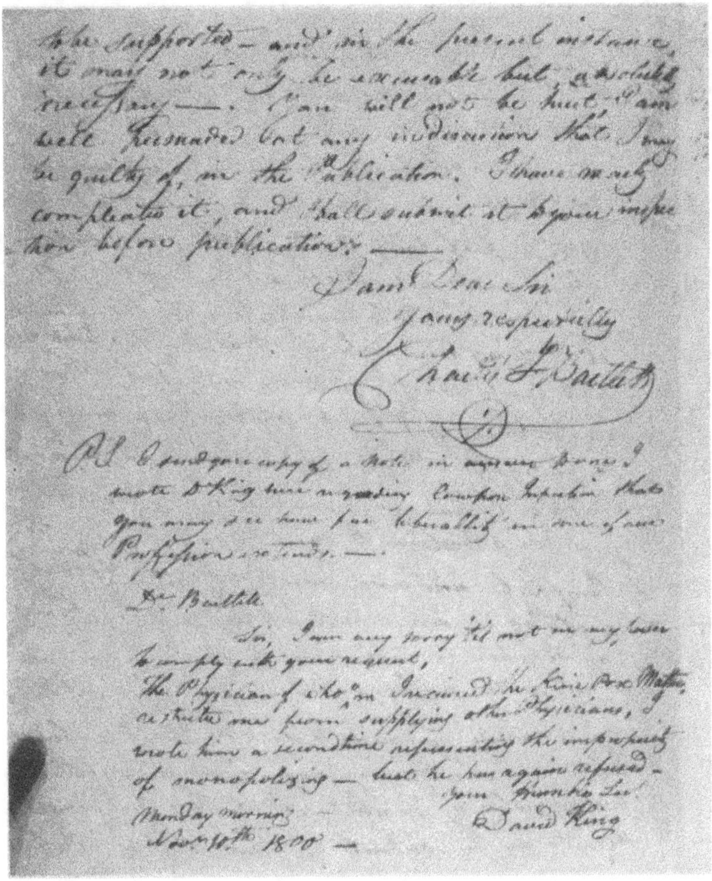

to be supported — and in the present instance, it may not only be excusable but, absolutely necessary —. You will not be hurt, I am well persuaded but any indiscretion that I may be guilty of, in the Publication. I have nearly compleated it, and shall submit it to your inspection before publication. —

I am Dear Sir
yours respectfully
Chas. F. Bartlett

P.S. I send you a copy of a Note in answer to one I wrote Dr King here regarding Cowpox Infection that you may see how far liberality in one of our Profession extends. —

Dr. Bartlett

Sir, I am very sorry 'tis not in my power to comply with your request,
The Physician of whom I received the Kine Pox Matter, restricts me from supplying other Physicians, I wrote him a second time representing the impropriety of monopolizing — but he has again refused —

Your Humble Ser.
David King

Monday morning
Nov. 10th 1800 —

Plate III. Letter from Charles F. Bartlett to Moses Brown, November 11, 1800, quoting letter from David King. (*Courtesy of Rhode Island Historical Society.*)

tained it from "a Doctor More, from Dummerstown"), and an additional amount "left with Mr. Hubbard by my friend, Captain —— of Windsor."[46]

Nor was Hedge the only physician who sought vaccine from Spalding. From Sanborntown, New Hampshire, Samuel Gerrish wrote on November 12 that the new inoculation was "the topic and rage" in his vicinity.

I think it probable [he continued] that I may inoculate a larger number, and make more, even under Doctor Waterhouse's restrictions, than to omit till Spring. That only, induces me to submit to his restrictions. I think that his method of restricting New Hampshire will answer his expectations but a short time. . . . If you cannot supply me in 12 to 15 days, be so good as to write, that I may procure it from some other quarter. Pudding Time I fear will be short.[47]

Down in Dedham, meanwhile, Dr. Nathaniel Ames, as we learn from his diary, had also obtained vaccine:

[October] 16 [1800]. . . . Took kine pox matter from P. Gay to innoculate.

19. Innoculated L. Parsons & Sam Gay Kine pox, which in six days works like small pox, headache, soreness of axilla, inflamed arm, &c: & prevents taking small pox. I have full faith. . . .

26. Sam Gay's cow pox works right, arm inflamed, soreness of axilla, &c.

31. Dr. Tudor of Orford, N.H. bro't Letter for B. Bissel, got kine pox matter. The people are yet infidels in the Blessing of Cow pox, or kine pox they cannot yet realize the security against Small pox.[48]

Further south, in Rhode Island, David King was unable to accommodate Dr. Charles F. Bartlett of Newport: "Sir," he wrote, "I am very sorry 'tis not in my power to comply with your request, The Physician of whom I received the Kine Pox Matter, restricted me from supplying other Physicians, I wrote him a second time representing the impropriety of monopolizing—but he has again refused." But a Dr. Wheaton of Providence "found means to procure the matter without Docr Waterhouse," and through the good offices of the Quaker philanthropist Moses Brown supplied the importunate Bartlett.[49]

III

THOUGH WATERHOUSE HAD RESTRICTED THE DISTRIBUTION of cowpox virus to profit from a monopoly, he also seems to have been genuinely worried that incompetent practitioners would obtain vaccine, or pseudo-vaccine, and give the new preventive a bad name. He set forth this reason in the *Centinel* on August 20 for not acceding to requests for the lymph, and he reprinted the statement in an appendix to his first pamphlet on vaccination, *A Prospect of Exterminating the Small-Pox*, which appeared about September 5.[50] In the latter he also pointed out that "there are some circumstances, which if not attended to critically, may bring the inoculation of this recently imported distemper into a temporary disrepute." The sources of spurious cowpox enumerated by Jenner, Waterhouse continued, were:

1st—That arising from pustules on the nipples, or udder of the cow, which pustules contain no specific virus.

2dly—From matter, (although originally possessing the specific virus,) which has suffered a decomposition, either from putrefaction, or from any other cause less obvious to the senses.

3dly—From matter taken from an ulcer in an *advanced stage*, which ulcer arose from a true cow-pox. . . . He [Jenner] . . . shews, that when the inoculated part has degenerated into an ulcer, the matter, although it may possess the power of inflaming the patient's arm, is nevertheless, void of that specific virus requisite to produce the genuine disease; and of course, incapable of securing the human system against the small-pox. . . .

Another circumstance, tending to discredit the idea of discarding the small-pox and substituting the kine-pox, is *mixing the two diseases together, and perhaps giving one for the other,* as we presume was done in some of the hospitals in London.[51]

After the monopoly had been breached, Waterhouse renewed and intensified his attack on spurious cowpox. In a letter to a country physician published in the *Massachusetts Mercury* of October 21 Waterhouse described "a vile traffic" in purported vaccine carried on from Boston to other towns. "What the matter is," he wrote, "I cannot tell, but of this I am certain, more has been sent into the country the last fortnight, than I have been able to collect from all my patients for a month, and I have innoculated [*sic*] twenty times as many as any man in the country." He feared that this "abominable practice" would bring the new discovery into disrepute:

> As this is *spurious* matter it never produces the requisite symptoms, and of course will not preserve a person from the small-pox, and one unfortunate instance would destroy all our exertions to extend far and wide one of the most important discoveries of modern times.[52]

At the end of the month an anonymous author came to Waterhouse's support. Everyone, he wrote, should uniformly "discountenance every attempt to propagate the disease, directed by avarice or assumed by ignorance, and unsupported by reason or propriety." Dr. Waterhouse's "unwearied exertions" to collect correct information, he continued, "are perfectly known in this neighborhood," while his testing his own children by variolation evinced his sincerity. Though the confusion of cowpox with smallpox in England had brought the new procedure into disrepute, "the united efforts of a respectable body of Physicians" had overcome this setback, and in Europe vaccination was "triumphing over every objection. . . ."

A subject of such importance [the author concluded], it behoves the public to watch with scrutinizing vigilance. For as in eight instances out of ten, the whole visible effect of the inoculated Kine-Pox is confined to the neighborhood of the incision, it is easy for any person, by any extraneous body inserted into the arm, to produce a sufficient inflamation [*sic*], to impose on those not acquainted with the appearances in the true disease. Thus while the deluded patient vainly supposes himself secured from the attacks of the Small-Pox, his imaginary safety leads him into situations where his life is endangered, and the properties of a disease, interesting to the world, are inveloped [*sic*] in doubt or brought into contempt by the crimes of avarice or the mistakes of ignorance.

The mischief arising from ignorance or artfulness in the management of this disease in Europe, have been sufficiently demonstrated by Dr. Waterhouse's publication on the subject; it therefore remains for Americans to encourage those gentlemen only, whose respectability of character places them beyond the charge of ignorance or suspicion.[53]

Unfortunately, however, Waterhouse's method of parceling out vaccine had rendered his motives suspect. Some practitioners believed that he warned against spurious cowpox in order to retain his monopolistic control. In the *Independent Chronicle* of November 3, a Bostonian, probably a physician, with biting sarcasm answered Waterhouse's letter to the country doctor. Since the new inoculation had become "considerably fashionable," he wrote, more cowpox matter had been "*sold* into the country, than could be made use of without involving the practitioner in inevitable disgrace and reproach. . . ." Yet "this 'abominable practice,' this 'vile traffic' " was among "the earliest exertions 'to extend far and wide one of the most important discoveries of modern times'!" Waterhouse, he implied, had failed to give those who purchased vaccine the instruction in its proper use which he should have provided. But "the vender," he supposed, might consider this of little consequence, provided he could "get rid of his commodity" at his own price.

Had Waterhouse not appealed, the letter writer continued, to

> the feelings of humanity, the pure principles of religion and the dearest interests of our country, . . . he would not have so justly incurred the imputation of insincerity and hypocrisy. Humanity, the principles of religion and the interests of our country have a powerful claim upon our best exertions; but it is an insult upon religion to attempt to enlist it in the cause of self-interest and sordid gain:—the Doctor had forgotten the scripture declaration—"*Ye cannot serve God and Mammon.*"

Whether there had been enormous exports of spurious cowpox virus from Boston, the writer professed not to know. Perhaps if Waterhouse would define the word "traffic," it could then be determined whether he was not himself the only one who had dealt in the "*vile traffic*" he so violently denounced. "We hope," the writer continued, "he has not combined *deception* in the quality of the Kine-Pox matter with extravagance of demand for it." And in a footnote he charged,

> It is a fact, and Dr. Waterhouse will not deny it, that the right of inoculating for the Kine-Pox disease has been actually districted *upon shares*, to certain physicians in the country, and for a series of years to come; this right has been *purchased* for one half or one third of the gain. Other physicians, I am told have paid, or conditioned to pay, the round sum of 150 dollars for the vaccine matter. These demands flow from the purest principles of *philanthropy*, and are authorised by the Doctor's unparalelled [*sic*] exertions to fix and establish the *credit* of the new discovery!!

Moreover, Waterhouse had declared spurious vaccine whose effect he knew nothing about—"a perfectability in the science which, it is presumed, no one had contemplated, and but few will aspire to." If Waterhouse really possessed

> a test by which he can infallibly determine the genuineness of the cow-pox matter, whether he has seen it or not, or knows at what time of the disease it was procured, he ought, for the instruction of his brethren of the faculty, and the good of the community, to let it be known:—humanity, religion, and our country, require it, and certainly the Doctor will not turn a deaf ear to these urgent calls.

Partly because Waterhouse's motives were questionable, and partly because of ignorance or, in some cases, knavery, large amounts of spurious cowpox were despite additional warnings [54] distributed through New England during the fall of 1800 and the following winter. Though Waterhouse's colorful account of this business [55] has often been repeated, it may not be amiss to mention some additional evidence. A Dr. Babbit of Sturbridge, for example, inoculated Cyrus Fay in December, 1800, with supposed vaccine obtained from a Connecticut physician.

> The matter [Fay later wrote] had a purulent cast, and was part of a shirt-sleeve worn during the plentiful discharge from the ulcerous state of the pustule. The inoculated arm appeared inflamed by the fourth day, and went on inflaming till about the 8th, when it became a running sore. . . . I concluded I had passed through the true disease, but as neither Dr. Babbit nor myself had ever seen the disease, we were at a loss to determine respecting the appearance of the arm. . . . I had thoughts of trying the experiment of the Small-Pox; had I unluckily done it, I should have added another spurious case, to perplex, confound and discourage the unexperienced Practitioner.[56]

Nor were some of the country folk above treating themselves. On December 8 James Parker of Shirley, Massachusetts, recorded in his diary, "David and Moody weare enocklated for the kin pox by Eastman . . ." Eight days later he noted, "I & Jam at evening put matter on our Arms in the Thine line [*sic*] or Cowpox." [57]

The most lamentable result of this malpractice occurred in Marblehead. Using virus that his seafaring son had taken from the arm of a sailor inoculated in London, Dr. Elisha Story on October 2 inoculated his daughter. Twelve days later, no symptoms having appeared, he concluded that the virus was bad and sent another son to Waterhouse to obtain a supply. On October 17, however, the girl broke out with cowpox, as Story supposed, so he did not use what Waterhouse had sent.[58] Actually she had smallpox, but Story, not realizing this, inoculated others, and before long the disease was rapidly spreading. Unable to control it, the town of Marblehead on November 10 decided on a general smallpox inoculation. In two days Story alone variolated more than a thousand persons. When the epidemic was over, sixty-eight persons had died. Meanwhile, about the time that Story's daughter first became ill, Waterhouse had vaccinated the son of Dr. John Drury, another Marblehead physician, to provide the latter with vaccine. Drury in turn treated some forty patients, all but one of whom later contracted smallpox. "However," the newspapers added, "it is only justice due to Dr. WATERHOUSE to acknowledge, that the two patients whom he inoculated with the Kine-Pox, were exempted from the general contagion. . . ." [59]

In his notice in the *Centinel* of August 20, 1800, Waterhouse had written that the preferred season for vaccination was from August to November. "Very cold weather," he asserted, "is unfavorable to the *Kine-pox*." But on September 25 he wrote Lyman Spalding, "I have no doubt but the inoculation will do very well all through the winter. I mean, at least, to try it." Toward the end of October, however, Waterhouse, like some other physicians, was running into difficulties. "By a late letter from him [Waterhouse]," wrote Josiah Bartlett to Spalding on October 30, "I find that the failure within *his* practice is equal to ours." [60] He was, as he later admitted, seriously perplexed, and to controvert the opinion of those who thought that in Marblehead cowpox had changed into smallpox, he wrote to the *Centinel* on November 14 that "If we are to judge of the force of the disease by the number of pustules, it certainly becomes milder as it recedes from the cow." It was well known, he added, that "cold diminishes the activity of febrile poisons," and it was obvious that the "vaccine poison" was less active now than it had been during the summer.[61]

On December 20 Waterhouse in another public letter stated that "For about two or three weeks in the month of November the matter seemed to have undergone a *deterioration* in my hands." He had had to inoculate several persons four or five times before the virus would take; with three or four he never could achieve success, and with some he was "still uncertain whether they have passed *fairly* through the disease or not." He was of the opinion, he continued, that "*the kine pox matter becomes milder as it recedes from the Cow*, and that in process of time it gets worn out, and . . . needs renewal." The fact that all the vaccine so far used in America "(some received at Ipswich excepted)" came from his stock lent support to the idea. He had therefore written to Jenner, Pearson, Woodville, and several other English physicians to suggest an arrangement whereby he might receive a monthly supply of vaccine "as *direct from the Cow* as possible" until cowpox was "naturalized" in America.[62] "Previously to which," he concluded, "I shall venture another communication entitled '*practical observations on the local appearance, symptoms, and mode of treating the kine-pox,'* which I hope to make through the medium of the public papers."[63] After this statement Waterhouse, who had already stopped vaccinating, retired from the field until March, when he received a new supply of good lymph from England.[64]

IV

THOUGH MANY PHYSICIANS WERE INOCULATING SPURIOUS cowpox during the fall of 1800, some were at least as competent as Waterhouse. Dr. Thomas Manning of Ipswich, who had imported his own lymph and soon supplied several other physicians, wrote a friend in Edinburgh on October 3 that cowpox was "rapidly becoming very general." There could be "no doubt of its universal diffusion," as fast as practitioners could obtain the virus. "Professor Waterhouse's occasional publications have done much in preparing the way for this comparatively benign substitute for the terror of the fair," he added, "and his practice has done still more in introducing it. I have inoculated many, all of whom either have done, or are doing extremely well." Moreover, at Manning's request the town of Ipswich on October 16 granted him permission to variolate ten persons who had had cowpox. The test was a complete success.[65] Josiah Bartlett of Charlestown, Massachusetts, vaccinated his son George on November 11, and "the appearance of his arm, and the symptoms, so fully corresponded with the plates and publications I had then seen, as to convince me, and others of my medical friends, that he had the *disease*." Their judgment was apparently correct, for two years later George was exposed to smallpox with impunity.[66] As late as January 20, 1801, James Jackson was still vaccinating, and with success, in the opinion of Drs. John Jeffries, John Warren, Thomas Welsh, and Aaron Dexter.[67]

Another known vaccinator was James Mann of Wrentham, several of whose patients were tested by variolation in 1800.[68] After signing a bond,[69] Mann received some thread from Waterhouse which he tried on twelve persons. This failing, he applied for more, and acquired enough to treat four patients. From their arms he supplied himself with additional lymph; "but uninformed with respect to the state of the pox, when the matter might be taken to communicate the disease, and having not read Dr. Jenner's Treatise at that time," he had to depend upon his own judgment, took the virus too late, and obtained only spurious cases. After many perplexing difficulties, Mann in time learned how to distinguish genuine cowpox from false, and when to take lymph from the vesicles of his patients. To a Boston physician—not Waterhouse—he wrote on November 8:

> I am happy that I have it in my power to correct my errors, and I am willing to acknowledge that I have been extremely ignorant respecting the progress and appearance of the specific disease of the Kine-Pox; and that I acquired the only accurate state of the genuine disease by an inspection of your patients, although I had had several, who I am well satisfied had passed regularly through it. And I moreover confess that I had not a divided idea, at what state of the disease, the virus should be taken for use, until I received information from you. I am now in the faith, that in no instance, we may have a spurious case, and since obtaining the matter in its limpid and transparent state; early inflammation, and superficial scabby arms have entirely disappeared.[70]

Though Waterhouse had provided Mann with vaccine, he had to learn from another physician how to use it properly.

Other incidents also show that Waterhouse was not the only, and perhaps not even the most careful, student of vaccination in Boston during this first year. The man who castigated his methods of distributing vaccine in the *Inde-*

pendent *Chronicle* of November 3 had remarked that the local physicians relied on Jenner's descriptions, believing that he "had *almost* as much knowledge of the nature and practice of the disease as any physician in the country." After the publication of Waterhouse's letter of December 20, another Boston physician also attacked Waterhouse's self-appointment as teacher of vaccination to America.[71] If cowpox inoculation, he wrote, required much nicer discernment than variolation, if no distinguishing criteria could with certainty be affixed to it, and "if in order to prevent spurious cases, a monthly importation of the vaccine-matter is necessary; then all our fair prospects . . . vanish at once. . . ." The idea of "some physicians," he continued, "that *'the Kine-Pox matter becomes milder as it recedes from the cow, and that in process of time it gets worn out,* . . .' cannot be admitted as a satisfactory solution of the difficulty. . . ." It was "in direct contrariety" to all that was known concerning the nature of contagion, and it could not be sustained "upon any established principles of analogy. . . ." Moreover, he wrote, "The idea is opposed to all the experience of European Physicians:—they positively assert, that the vaccine matter is equally specific and efficacious after having passed through an indefinite number of patients as when taken immediately from the cow."

After presenting his own (incorrect) theory on the cause of the current difficulties, the writer suggested that "A collection of facts from the different Physicians in this town" on this subject was "a very desirable object, as promotive of public good;" but he would pause for now "and wait until favored with the promised publication of '*Practical Observations*, &c.,' " in which he hoped to find all doubtful points and difficulties fully and fairly considered, and the true criteria of cowpox ascertained. But he also hoped that the Marblehead practitioners would communicate their observations. "Facts from this quarter," he wrote, "must have more weight in fixing the public sentiment than any thing that has yet appeared in this country." Finally, this Boston physician enclosed a letter "replete with real facts and judicious remarks" for publication in the newspaper—the letter from James Mann quoted earlier.

Obviously the author did not feel that Waterhouse, for all his talk, had as yet contributed significantly to the discussion of the new technique. It seems possible that Waterhouse sent an extract of a letter that he had received from Mann to the *Centinel* a few days later partly to show that he too was still the valued friend, correspondent, and confidant of the Wrentham physician.[72]

Then, a month later, in a communication to the *Centinel*, James Jackson reported on his experiences. Although thousands of English cases attested to the preventive power of cowpox, any apparent deviation from the general principle, he noted, should be fully and publicly recorded. "It is also proper for me to declare to those whom I have inoculated for the cow-pox," he added, "that my confidence in it is not so perfect as it once was." He then reported in detail upon the case of a man named Wheelock whom he had vaccinated in October, who had been inoculated with smallpox in January, and who had developed symptoms that led Jackson to believe that he might have contracted the disease. Those who knew him, Jackson continued, would readily conceive "that I have not witnessed these circumstances without mortification. But it will not save my feelings to conceal the facts. It is more pleasing to me to give my evidence in favor of the truth even against an opinion of which I have been an advocate." The case, he urged, should be independently examined by other gentlemen of the faculty. Should they find him in error, he remarked, "no person will be more gratified than myself." He would not say for sure, he concluded, that Wheelock had had smallpox. But his case had "excited in my mind doubts, which I thought I should never find there." At the most it could only prove "that the cow-pox does not always preserve the subject of it from the small-pox; but this is an inconsistency in the operations of nature to which we should not give full credit without the clearest evidence." [73]

An honor to Jackson's candor and modesty, this statement also gave at least two other doctors an opportunity to differ publicly with his diagnosis and to express their confidence in vaccination. The experiment, wrote one, "does not by any means demonstrate, even in that case, that the small-pox did actually supervene." Similar cases had occurred, he continued, without leading the attending physician to believe that the effect was more than a local inflammation. Though willing to admit his error should "uncontrovertible evidence" stare him in the face, Jackson's communication gave him "no reason to change an opinion which has been established upon actual experiment made by himself that the Cow pox renders the human system unsusceptible to the *small-pox*." [74]

With this view another practitioner agreed:

Dr. J's personal opportunity in *England* to gain a full knowledge of the true characteristics of Cow-pox, no medical gentlemen would be so uncandid as to suppose he could have left on his mind a single doubt whether his patient had the disease. While we render the Dr. the just praise due for the accuracy of his statement, his liberality, and love of truth, we trust he will not take offence, should we differ from him in opinion that doubts which previous to this case never have existed, ought to be entertained of the efficacy of cow-pox, and that the doubts as to small pox, in which the case is enveloped, are *alone* sufficient to confirm, rather than weaken his original opinion, and ought not to excite in the public mind, prejudices, already too indiscriminate, against what we have the fullest ground of belief, will be found most essential to the happiness of the world at large.[75]

The incident also brought a tactful letter from Manning, which Jackson transmitted to the newspaper:

Of those, who have been inoculated in this vicinity with vaccine matter from the same source as your's, ten have since been inoculated with variolous matter, and exposed to its infection. None of them had the least degree of symptomatic fever; several had their arms more or less inflamed, and one of them had two or three pustules.

Upon the whole the balance of experimental evidence appears at present in favor of the vaccine disease, and while this is the case I think it entitled to our undiminished confidence.[76]

V

While awaiting new vaccine from England during the winter of 1801, Waterhouse seems to have concluded that his original method of distribution had been a serious mistake. After his supply had been reestablished in March, 1801, he acted upon different principles. Receiving requests for lymph from unknown correspondents in the South, he sent it instead to Thomas Jefferson, who had already expressed an interest in the new preventive. The President in turn supplied many physicians throughout the South and as far north as Philadelphia with their first genuine cowpox virus. No hint of monopoly or recompense intruded upon these negotiations. They were highly creditable to Waterhouse's character and professional skill, as well as to Jefferson's humanity and ingenuity.[77]

In Boston, the first result of this new attitude appeared in the *Centinel* on April 1, 1801. After announcing the receipt of good vaccine from England, Waterhouse wrote that when he had commenced the new inoculation in America, he had had "special reasons for wishing to confine the trials, for awhile, to three or four practitioners." Accordingly he had given the virus to three physicians "long experienced in the inoculated small-pox, even before the disease had gone through my own family." But since these considerations no longer existed in their full force, he would "adopt a different conduct" and "try to avoid the blunder of dispersing it to so many inexperienced persons at a distance."

Recent information from England, Waterhouse continued, confirmed his assertion that a person who had undergone cowpox was secure from smallpox. Yet, since the accidents at Marblehead and the Wheelock case had created doubts, vaccination should be tested by variolation, as it had been in England and on the Continent. He wished now, he wrote, principally

> to suggest the idea of a VACCINE INSTITUTION in *Boston*, or its neighborhood for the inoculation of the poor *gratis*, and so arranged as to admit of the trial of the small-pox *after* the kine-pox, and that this institution should be *immediately* under the direction of AGED and EXPERIENCED practitioners, and *remotely* under the controul of the *Board of Health*.

Pointing out in support of this proposal that a general smallpox inoculation caused many deaths and universal business distress, a Bostonian called upon the wealthy to found such an institution and pay the cost of testing vaccinated persons. "Interest should induce our merchants to take this measure," he concluded, "and every other, which may introduce a general inoculation for the vaccine disease; as otherwise the town must ere long be shut up for a general variolous inoculation." By the end of May subscription papers were available in State Street insurance offices for those who wished to contribute.[78] But the only public response of the "aged and experienced practitioners," who had heard of the bonds and knew that Waterhouse had monopolized the practice in Boston as long as he could, was that implied in a letter from Jackson published on April 8, in which he announced the receipt of some "cow pox matter" from London. He and some other Boston physicians were vaccinating all poor applicants gratis, he noted, and no doubt all those interested in the introduction of the new preventive would do the same. "While the poor are benefitted by this arrangement," he explained, "the physician will find a compensation in the constant supply of fluid matter, on which depends very much the certainty of success in inoculating for this disease." [79]

Four days earlier, Waterhouse had met Isaac Rand, the president of the Massachusetts Medical Society, on a street in Boston. He told Waterhouse that the Society had just received some vaccine which had been ordered from London in January, that it had been distributed among a few of the members but had failed in their hands, and that he feared it would fail in his own.[80] On the following day, April 5, Waterhouse sent to Rand what he later described as an official letter, enclosing some lymph. Since he had made arrangements for a monthly supply from England, he wrote, he hoped to be able to afford the Society a never failing source.

> Having imported a new disease, or to speak more properly, a new remedy [Waterhouse continued], I am, as may be supposed, ambitious to diffuse its benefits through our land, but am entirely at a loss for the just and proper method; on which account I feel disposed to submit the matter to the advice and direction of the Massachusetts Medical Society. I acceeded [*sic*] to the written proposals of a number of practitioners, at a distance, the past season; but that mode was never wholly to my satisfaction. In order then to give satisfaction to the faculty, to the public and to myself, I wish now to place myself under the direction and advice of the Society.

Waterhouse then suggested that since neither he nor the Society had been able to obtain an accurate account of the Marblehead epidemic, it might be advisable to appoint a committee to make the necessary investigation on the spot.[81] It is unfortunate that Waterhouse, whose proposal was sincere,[82] sent the letter to Rand rather than to the Corresponding Secretary, to whom, as an official letter, it should have been addressed. For Rand considered it personal, and never brought it to the Society's attention.[83]

When the Council met on April 29, Waterhouse came to Boston and personally urged various members to appoint a committee of inquiry.[84] The Council, acceding, picked Waterhouse, President Rand, and Vice-President Warren. When the day planned for the trip arrived, however, Warren and Rand, being both unable to go, dispatched a servant to tell Waterhouse (they subsequently averred), but Waterhouse apparently never received the message and as a result found himself alone in Marblehead. Warren informed his colleague a few days later that he had been called to an urgent case, and Rand immediately wrote to the Society explaining why he had been detained; yet Waterhouse conceived that he had been intentionally left in the lurch. Though the committee never officially reported, the Council decided on June 3 that the receipt of four letters on the epidemic "prevented the necessity of any further attention to that subject." [85]

Thus in the spring of 1801 the Boston profession had ignored Waterhouse's suggestion for a vaccine institution. The Massachusetts Medical Society, never having received his letter to Rand, had failed to act upon it. And the President and Vice-President of the Society, Waterhouse believed, had purposely left him to face the angry citizens of Marblehead alone. A contentious person by nature, Waterhouse understandably felt bitter.

After waiting in vain for an answer to his request for advice and direction, Waterhouse late in June reverted to the newspapers. Since people were less willing to believe events occurring at a distant time or place, he argued, it was essential to publicize all American cases that demonstrated the efficacy of vaccination. It had been hoped, he went on, that "some *Medical* or *Philosophical Society*" would act as a center for collecting and disseminating such information. "But as a propitious season is fast passing away, without any prospect of such an advantage, Dr. WATERHOUSE is constrained to adopt a more diminutive plan, and to go on in this business as he began it—*alone*." Calling for case reports from practitioners who had successfully "put the kine pox to the *test* of the small pox," he concluded by requesting printers throughout the nation to republish his letter, "and *Patriotism* will carry it to their credit." [86]

During the rest of 1801 and throughout 1802 Waterhouse performed yeoman service. He distributed both lymph and instructions gratuitously not only to Jefferson, but also to Valentine Seaman in New York,[87] to the United States Army, and to many other practitioners. So extensive did his correspondence become, that in April, 1802, to save the labor of handwriting, he reprinted some concise directions which Jenner had recently sent him.[88] Waterhouse also kept up his propaganda barrage in the *Centinel* and other Boston newspapers. He sent information on proper techniques; warned against spurious cases and inexperienced or lay practitioners; investigated reports of smallpox following cowpox; transmitted accounts of the tested success of the new inoculation; relayed information from New York, Philadelphia, and England on the progress of vaccination; and drew up a long list of cases in an attempt to prove that the protective power of cowpox lasted for life.[89]

At the same time, Waterhouse was not the only medical man promoting vaccination in the Boston newspapers. In the *Palladium*, for example, "A Physician" sharply answered "A Tradesman" who hoped the town would allow a general smallpox inoculation in Boston during the summer of 1801.[90] One Cyrus Fay supported Waterhouse's contention that many had used spurious matter.[91] From Hallowell, Maine, came the report of a previously vaccinated man who had been variolated four times without effect,[92] and from Portsmouth, New Hampshire, an account of a successful public experiment by Lyman Spalding.[93] In October, 1801, both the *Palladium* and the *Chronicle* reprinted a certificate by Asaph Coleman, a Connecticut inoculator, that he had been unable to give smallpox to several persons vaccinated by Dr. Samuel Cooley of Bolton.[94] The following month the *Chronicle* carried the news that cowpox had been found in American cattle by three country physicians in southern New England,[95] and the *Palladium* printed reports in February and June, 1802, of the successful experiments of Nathaniel Miller of Franklin, Massachusetts.[96] In August, 1802, the *Centinel* published a letter from Dr. John G. Coffin of Boston describing the resistance of several persons in Maine to smallpox infection following vaccination. "This statement," he wrote, ". . . may be esteemed an addition of some importance to that weight of other evidence which has produced a conviction in my mind, that . . . vaccination . . . destroys the susceptibility [to smallpox] . . . for the remainder of life." [97]

The newspapers also informed their readers of Jefferson's progress with the lymph that Waterhouse had sent, of his endorsement of the procedure, and of his donation of the blessing to Little Turtle and other visiting Indians.[98] They extracted accounts from books and other journals of the advance of vaccination in England, France, Sweden, and Russia, as well as in New York, Baltimore, and Charleston.[99] From local citizens, too, came occasional messages. One urged doubters to read C. R. Aikin's *Concise View* on cowpox, which was reprinted in Charlestown in 1801; another warned against apparent failures due to spurious cases; and a third sent a statistical table of seven eighteenth-century smallpox epidemics in Boston to emphasize the benefits of the new preventive.[100]

Nevertheless, many citizens remained skeptical. Some were no doubt innately suspicious of anything new. Others probably considered the whole business a scheme pushed by the doctors for their own profit. Rumors persisted that persons who had been vaccinated had subsequently been infected with smallpox, and if these were exposed as cases of spurious cowpox, they nevertheless lent credence to a belief that the new inoculation was so difficult and uncertain in practice that variolation remained the only sure way to acquire immunity. And the old procedure was further reinforced by the assertion that the protective power of even a properly performed vaccination would last but a few years.[101]

Though rarely expressed in public print, the rationale of the opposition was in part exposed by Dr. William Aspinwall. After Waterhouse had first successfully tested his family in that physician's hospital in August, 1800, the inoculator reportedly exclaimed, "this new Inoculation of yours, is no sham. As a man of humanity, I rejoice in it; although it will take from me a handsome annual income." [102] Describing these events in September, 1800, Waterhouse generously acknowledged that he could not have completed his tests without Aspinwall's assistance. The latter, he wrote, "met these experiments, which *apparently* militate at present, with his interest, with a candor, and ingenuousness much to his praise." His conduct had done "honor to his liberality as a practitioner, and to his patriotism as a citizen." [103]

On October 1, 1801, however, to an advertisement of his hospital in the *Chronicle*, Aspinwall appended a notice that "Six persons who were inoculated with the KINE-POX last year, and supposed to have had that disease, have been inoculated at the above said Hospital, the present year, and five of the six have had the SMALL-Pox perfectly." [104] The first reaction, which appeared in the next issue of the same paper, was an observation by "A correspondent" that the "five persons who had been *supposed* to have gone through the Kine-Pox" were not, as some had inferred, Waterhouse's patients: "The fact is six of Dr. Waterhouse's family, and another person he sent in this summer, and which Dr. Aspinwall inoculated, *all withstood the small-pox.*" [105]

Soon after, Waterhouse published a letter in the *Palladium* reiterating this point. Furthermore, he wrote, he had supplied the vaccine for only one of the five, an employee whom Aspinwall had himself vaccinated.[106] When Aspinwall's advertisement next appeared in the *Chronicle,* it was immediately succeeded by another statement from the Cambridge professor. He had applied to Aspinwall for an explanation, he declared, "and having waited ten days for an answer, have concluded that he does not mean to give one." Had Aspinwall added a note that none of the reported failures were Waterhouse's patients, he continued, it would have "*obviated the uneasiness of some parents, and added one more to the obligations I felt myself under to Dr. Aspinwall.*" And, he remarked, "*I still hope the Dr. will give to the public all the circumstances of the inoculations mentioned in his* too concise *advertisement.*" [107] Privately, Waterhouse's reaction was considerably more acrid. On October 20 he wrote to Matthias Spalding, a former student then in London, that Aspinwall, whose "candor and liberality was all affectation," had "shown his teeth" by inoculating those "*whom he knew had never gone fairly through the disease,*" and then advertising the result. "It was just his harvest time," Waterhouse asserted, "it staggered several who were balancing between the S. pox and kine pox, and occasioned perhaps

20 or 30 to go into his hospital. He gives out that the K. pox will preserve from infection for a few months *but no longer*." [108]

Soon after this outburst, Aspinwall named the six persons and presented some of the details relating to their vaccination. As to Isaac Sawyer, the one whom he had himself treated the previous November, he claimed that "Whether he had the *genuine* Kine-pox, or *spurious*, the matter with which he was inoculated, was received by me directly from Dr. WATERHOUSE, and immediately used." Waterhouse, he continued, had supplied him with vaccine four times, with which he had inoculated thirteen persons, "and on some of them it had no effect—on some it produced very sore arms, and one only, the *Kine-pox*, less equivical [*sic*] than that of Sawyer." [109] Less directly, through the remarks of "A Friend," Aspinwall had already offered the reason for his original publication: while professing entire confidence in the protective powers of cowpox, he contended that there was "*less certainty in its taking*, than in the SMALL-POX;" he was not convinced that there would be a gain in "discarding one to adopt the other." He did wish for "a fair trial and candid experiment." [110]

Apparently mollified, Waterhouse thanked Aspinwall for his explanatory statement. "It is by such open and candid discussions," he continued, "that we may expect to come at the truth. . . ." After giving further details and some notes on the sources of spurious vaccination, he disavowed any intention to reflect on Aspinwall. He was, Waterhouse wrote, more attached to the old inoculation, with which he had been so successful, than to the new. This was natural, Waterhouse explained: "He is like other men attached to his interest, but I believe he is attached to the great cause of humanity more." His only sentiments towards Aspinwall, Waterhouse concluded, were "those of respect and esteem." [111] Nor were these remarks intended solely for public consumption. The following spring Waterhouse wrote to Matthias Spalding that he hoped John Ring would "not name Aspinwall in terms that may hurt his feelings. I have many apologies to make for him," he added. "There are hundreds worse than he is in the opposition. His hospital is his own property and he will lose 1500 guineas a year by it." [112]

Meanwhile, during the year ending April 1, 1801, the Boston Board of Health had removed some sixty sailors suffering with smallpox from vessels arriving at the port. Though several persons had broken out with the disease in the town itself during the fall of 1800, the Board had controlled the incipient epidemic by taking most of the sick to the quarantine hospital on Rainsford Island and confining the rest in their homes.[113] When another case appeared in Boston in May, 1802, many neighbors, terrified despite the health officials' prompt isolation of the patient, hastened to Aspinwall's hospital.[114] Though the Board of Health had in June, 1801, rejected James Jackson's request for permission to test some of the people he had vaccinated, alleging that "the avocations of the Board would not permit that attention which the plan proposed by Dr. JACKSON required," [115] Waterhouse forcefully memorialized the Board on May 31, 1802, to undertake a convincing public experiment. Accepting his proposal, the Board, after consulting James Lloyd, Isaac Rand, Samuel Danforth, John Warren, Charles Jarvis, and John Jeffries, as well as Waterhouse, obtained the town's permission to perform the smallpox inoculations at some spot outside the peninsula. On August 16 nineteen young volunteers were vaccinated at the health office and a week later the examining physicians pronounced them "fit subjects for the Experiment contemplated." After erecting a temporary hospital on Noddle's Island, the Board secured fresh smallpox virus in November from a Falmouth inoculator and subjected the nineteen, along with another lad vaccinated two years previously, both to variolation and to contact with two unprotected controls who were inoculated to prove that the smallpox matter was active. The test was a complete success. Finally, the Board published a detailed report in mid-December with a supporting statement signed by eleven physicians and urged the public to use the new preventive.[116] "This decisive experiment," Waterhouse wrote soon after, ". . . has fixed forever the practice of the new inoculation in Massachusetts." [117]

VI

WHILE BENJAMIN WATERHOUSE'S EFFORTS DURING AND after 1801 to diffuse the benefits of vaccination were presumably sincere, he was not wholly candid about his operations during the summer and fall of 1800. Recognizing, perhaps, that his own approach had in fact fostered vaccination quackery and a speculative, mercenary attitude, and that his efforts to build a monopoly ill accorded with his pretensions to philanthropy; knowing that he could no longer in any event retain exclusive control over the supply of vaccine; and probably realizing that his actions, if widely known, would not only reflect upon his own character but also tend to discredit vaccination itself, Waterhouse sought to explain away or conceal his own culpability.

To Lettsom, for example, he wrote on April 6, 1801, that he had asked the Massachusetts Medical Society for their opinion as to the best way to distribute the cowpox virus, "for last year it got into the hands of speculators and quacks, notwithstanding every effort of mine to prevent it, which one of my friends at Bath [John Haygarth?] seems to have misunderstood." [118]

Writing to President Timothy Dwight of Yale on March 23, 1801, Waterhouse was more emphatic. So insistent was the demand for vaccine, he explained, that he had found it necessary to give up his original plan for "a rigid set of experiments," and he went, he feared, "into the opposite extreme." The clamor, he continued, "had a doubly bad effect, which I did not at first foresee, but which I was sensible of when they began to apply for it from Connecticut, which accounts for my refusal of them. But the motive of my refusal was misconstrued and they obtained some sort of matter elsewhere." When failures resulted, those who had formed "*extravagant* expectations" were the first to denounce vaccination as a "delusion" and "mere money speculation!" No wonder accidents occurred when a practitioner would even encourage children to treat each other, just to destroy a rival's business. "Contrast this abominable conduct," he wrote, "with the extreme care and caution exercised in *England* and lately at *Paris* in this new innoculation." [119]

Even more illuminating is a letter to Jefferson which Waterhouse sent on October 1, 1801, just after hearing that the President had successfully established vaccination in Washington and parts of Virginia. "Avarice, rivalship, and mistrust," he remarked, had attended the introduction of the practice in New England. Some physicians had ridden night and day to reach Cambridge ahead of their professional brethren, and others claiming to be his agents had endangered the lives of the people by hawking spurious matter. Six New Hampshire practitioners, he asserted, "absolutely new districted the State, and then applied to me for the matter, and offering me their conjoint bonds to give me a fourth part of all that were inoculated by them & their subordinates! so that before I well knew the spirit & extent of the plan, I found myself the centre of a vile speculation." But by sending the virus to Jefferson, Waterhouse wrote, he had forestalled similar events in the South.[120]

At a later date, April 2, 1803, Waterhouse explained in a letter to Major Daniel Jackson his refusal to accept any pay for sending vaccine and instructions for treating soldiers. In promoting this procedure, he wrote, he had had "*more powerful motives than private emolument.*" But since the work was inevitably attended with considerable expense, he decided, after consulting "leading medical and clerical characters," to impose a "small assessment" on those practitioners who sought instruction and vaccine solely for their own profit. Gladly would he have avoided this "tax," but "not being a man of property, *it was impossible.*" To medical societies, vaccine institutions, and "*influential characters,*" however, he had "*unremittingly and gratuitously*" distributed both the lymph and written instructions. "Supplying the means for inoculating the Battalion under your command," Waterhouse concluded, "I can consider in no other light than that of a PUBLIC BENEFIT, and when considered in this view I have invariably refused any pecuniary consideration whatever." [121] Most of this appears to be true. But it is hard to think of "$150 for a district not containing more inhabitants than Kittery," [122] or one quarter of the profits of a year's practice, as a "small assessment."

Despite these disclaimers, the story of the bonds refused to die. On July 21, 1802, Waterhouse wrote a letter to the *Centinel* contradicting the assertion that vaccination conferred only temporary protection:

> After the absurd doctrine respecting the *short duration* of the efficacy of the kine-pock, is no longer urged [he concluded], there is but one other scheme to which the enemies of the new inoculation can have recourse for effecting its disgrace, and that is throwing it into the hands of improper persons. . . . I should not have glanced at this subject at this time, were not the same practices now going forward in a town close by *Boston,* where from the delusive offers of inoculating *gratis,* or for a very small fee, people have been induced to receive the disease from persons not qualified to judge between the *true* and the *spurious* pustule; the consequence has already been that children have followed the example and inoculated one another. The result will be, some of these imprudent people will go into the neigh-

bouring hospital, take the small-pox, and then the odium will as usual revert to me, because the matter used was taken from my patients. I therefore feel it no more than justice to myself, (considering the pains I have taken to mature this business) and a duty I owe to the public, to notice this conduct of ignorance and presumption.[123]

Two men thought this letter aimed specifically at them. One obtained a private explanation with which he was satisfied.[124] The other, who had something of a temper, demanded a public disavowal, and in the next issue of the *Centinel* appeared a notice signed by Waterhouse denying any allusion to John C. Howard: ". . . from my knowledge of Mr. HOWARD's classical and medical education," he added, "it cannot be supposed that I meant to rank him with the ignorant and presumptuous." [125]

Had Waterhouse refrained from further personal observations, this would undoubtedly have ended the matter. But on August 2 he embroidered his first brief acknowledgment with another newspaper statement. In the earlier note, he addressed the editor, he "neglected to mention" an important point:

Some time last May I inoculated Mr. John Howard's *child* at Dorchester, WITH A VIEW *to shew him the disease and* FOR THE EXPRESS PURPOSE *of giving him the genuine vaccine virus to make experiments with, agreeably to a promise I had long made him.*—This *forgotten* fact speaks for itself.—In further justice to myself I feel now free to declare that it was only since that publication, that I was acquainted with the extent of the inoculations performed by a *Merchant* and a *Lawyer* in *Dorchester* and *Roxbury*. Had I have known it, I should hardly have been so forgetful of propriety as to have advertised the gentlemen, but seeing I was the *originator* of the experiments in *Dorchester* as well as in *Roxbury*, I should probably have taken the liberty to interpose my friendly advice, and that for the following reasons, which I deem sufficiently important to VACCINATION, *at this period*, to merit a place in your paper.

First, all *gratuitous* inoculations on an extensive scale should be commenced and conducted by a PUBLIC VACCINE INSTITUTION. . . .

Second, young physicians, (not to mention those who are not physicians) have universally conceived more lightly of this new inoculation than is consistent with the nature of things. . . . I fear lest this new inoculation should not be commenced and *tested* by persons sufficiently experienced in the kine-pock and in the SMALL-POX. Have not occurrences in own [*sic*] country justified this fear? How has it happened that of between 20 and 30 young Doctors to whom I have given the vaccine virus, have almost all of them within a few months got a ground and given up the business? They found as they went on, that this *very simple business*, required more attention than they at first imagined. . . .

As to gentlemen acting out of the line of their profession, . . . Has not a disregard to these lines of "*demarkation*" given origin, in the case before us, to a practice among mechanics and day labourers . . . ? [126]

It is hardly surprising that Howard, who, although not then in general practice, was a regularly educated physician,[127] felt called upon to reply. He had been willing, he wrote, "tacitly to acquiesce" in Waterhouse's first acknowledgment, but his new communication required some further observations. "Dr. WATERHOUSE insinuates," he noted, "that I had requested him to inoculate my child with the Vaccine virus with a view to show me the disease." To be sure, he had asked Waterhouse for some lymph, "but a long time having elapsed, without obtaining it," he had resorted to another physician, "who had more than once furnished Dr. W. and who promised to supply me at any time." Since he had frequently loaned Waterhouse publications on vaccination, Howard continued, he had considered himself authorized to make such an application "without incurring the hazard of a tax on my gratitude, which I might hereafter be unwilling or unable to pay. Although a *merchant*, I was not then aware that this *virus* had been, and still was a *subject for traffick and barter*." Some time later Waterhouse called and without Howard's knowledge or consent insisted upon vaccinating his child.

Furthermore, Howard rejoined, he had "positive and respectable evidences" to prove that Waterhouse was before his first "exceptionable publication" fully aware of the extent of Howard's practice in Dorchester. Indeed, Waterhouse had "expressed much surprize and dissatisfaction at my procedure; and more than insinuated that I was not competent to the business I had undertaken." Had it not been for this fact, Howard wrote, he would not have bothered to demand an explanation. But he conceived it due to those whom he had treated to remove all doubts "which any malevolent insinuations of my incapacity" might have aroused. He continued:

It was my good fortune to have been in *England* when the happy discovery of *Vaccine Inoculation* was first announced by Doct. JENNER. At once impressed with the importance of the subject I soon felt an interest in its success. From this early date my confidence in the efficacy of the Vaccine Inoculation has not been impaired; and I have been sedulous to inform myself of its progress by the regular importation of most of the publications on the subject. Deriving my information then from such sources, it can hardly be supposed that I sought any instructions from Dr. W. although he seemed to pretend to a superior knowledge of the disease, and wished to secure an exclusive practice in it. Time will discover if this were the best mode for making this invaluable discovery the most generally useful; and whether its blessings were best to be diffused by imparting the matter for inoculation generally to those only, who would give bonds for a proportion of the pecuniary profits resulting from its use, or by selling it like the *nostrums of quackery and empiricism.*

Until public skepticism had been overcome, Howard believed, gratuitous vaccination was the most likely means of extending the practice. It hardly seemed probable that this would endanger the "regular and honest profits" of the medical profession.[128] To this letter Waterhouse at that time made no public reply.[129]

Once again, in the fall of 1802, the bonds were mentioned. During the course of the experiment conducted by the Board of Health, Isaac Rand alluded to them in a private conversation with Waterhouse, "and pointed out to him what I [Rand] thought if the report was true might extricate him from the injurious consequences of it to his character." Waterhouse, however, denied the whole charge, and the matter rested.[130] In December the health officials presented their report, and shortly thereafter Waterhouse published his second volume on vaccination, *A Prospect of Exterminating the Small Pox Part II.*[131] During the next few years occasional references to the man and his work, none derogatory, appeared in the *Centinel,* but Waterhouse himself retired from his public literary labors in this cause.[132]

VII

Praised by Jenner and Ring, honored by physicians and laymen in other American cities, acclaimed in the newspapers of his own locality, Waterhouse might well have felt content in contemplating the contribution he had made to the welfare of the nation. But such was not the nature of the man. The real and fancied slights that he had received from the profession in Boston continued to rankle, and in 1806 he sent to the *Centinel* a slashing attack upon the Massachusetts Medical Society and a spirited defense against the imputation of personal profit-seeking.

After presenting in familiar phraseology his own version of the introduction of vaccination, his warnings against spurious cases, and the reaction which followed the Marblehead epidemic, he recounted his troubles with the Society. Understanding that the vaccine which it had received from London had failed, he wrote, he sent some of his own and at the same time requested the appointment of a committee to investigate the Marblehead affair. But the other members of the committee, after making every arrangement, "left me alone to encounter, for aught they knew, the resentment of an enraged populace." The public should know, he thought, how he had been treated by those who should have offered him every encouragement.

So much was I engaged in pushing vaccination as a *public benefit*, and so little avaricious of personal profit or reputation, that in 1801, when I had obtained a new recruit of matter from *England*, and when my practice was free from spurious cases, I offered to put myself under the advice and controul [*sic*] of the

Massachusetts Medical Society. I wished to make them the central point to which every thing relating to this new inoculation might be reflected, and every where extend its power of illumination. But an illiberal construction was put on my application, and I was compelled to go on in this business, as I began it, ALONE.

Soon after, he reported, he again felt it his duty to warn the public against ignorant pretenders and spurious cases. But "the most illiberal part of the profession" attributed this "disinterested advice" to a desire to "create doubts and fears, and to raise difficulties and perplexities, in order to confine the business to my own hands." Despite a resulting abusive publication and anonymous threats, he continued to devote all his time and attention to the promulgation of the truth. Knowing the physicians of Boston would not follow his lead, he had memorialized the Board of Health to make a convincing experiment, which this "*standing committee of humanity*" had carried through to a triumphant conclusion.[133]

When the Massachusetts Medical Society convened for its annual meeting in June, this attack not unnaturally occasioned some remarks. Directed to inquire into the matter, the Counsellors appointed a committee of investigation headed by Dr. William Eustis (who was, incidentally, by far the most prominent Jeffersonian-Republican politician among the members of the profession in Boston [134]). Seeking explanations, Eustis called upon Waterhouse, who replied with a "letter of defiance": [135]

Sir, I have been too sick ever since the day you called on me, to attend to any business whatever; even this is written by repeated efforts, and is merely to thank you for your kindness; and I think I reciprocate it, when I say that I trust the gentlemen of the Medical Society will play their game with caution, when I assure them that *I have some trump cards in my hand*.[136]

Thereupon the committee and the Counsellors, after searching the Society's files, drew up their report.[137]

They could find no evidence, they wrote, that Waterhouse had sent vaccine to the Society or had offered to put himself under its control. Probably Waterhouse had, "after a certain period," given the virus to individual members; that they had also supplied him was "unquestionably true." If Waterhouse did propose to any members of the Society to place himself under its direction, the Society had taken no order upon the subject, and therefore could not be charged with want of liberality. Getting to the heart of the matter, they declared:

> The assertion of Dr. W. that he was pursuing vaccination as a public benefit, and not for personal profit, does not accord with a notorious fact, viz. that until the virus had been received from *Europe* through other channels, he kept the matter in his own hands, excepting that it was imparted to those, who were ready to give him bonds for a pecuniary remuneration, proportionable to the profits of the business. When Dr. W. intimates that other physicians doubted the success of the inoculation, ought he not in candor to state, at the same time, his own embarrassments, arising from many spurious cases among his own patients?

The fact that the Society had sent to England for lymph in January, 1801, the committee reported, proved that it was not indifferent to the diffusion of vaccination; moreover, this importation did not fail, as Waterhouse himself well knew. "Nor is there better foundation for his attempt to propagate the opinion," they added, "that physicians here were averse to the introduction of the vaccine disease; for no where has it been better received by medical men." Since Waterhouse had been informed as soon as practicable of the reasons why the other members of the Marblehead committee had been unable to go, they were, they concluded, "at a loss to conceive, what motives could suggest, and what excuse can palliate the intimation of insincerity on the part of the committee." [138]

Obviously awaiting this opening, Waterhouse then produced his "*trump cards*," the letter he had written to Rand in April, 1801. What shall we think of a Society, he demanded, "who shall so conduct, as to allow a simple individual to meet them publicly with such a flat contradiction as is this *official* letter?" Though Rand would no doubt claim it was private, the attention given to the request for a Marblehead committee proved that the Society had seen the letter and treated the rest of it with "silent neglect." [139]

Taking up the cudgels for the Society, an anonymous Fellow (probably John Collins Warren and James Jackson [140]) returned blow for blow.

> It is with reluctance [he began] I call the attention of the public to Dr. WATERHOUSE. They I know are fatigued and disgusted with the frequent displays of himself which *he* has made. Few persons need be informed of his impotence in every thing but vain-boasting of himself, and dark and artful insinuations respecting others. But continual misrepresentations must be exposed.[141]

Backed by statements from Rand and others, the Fellow pointed out in this and subsequent letters that Rand had indeed considered the letter private and that the Society, never having seen it, could not be charged with illiberality. That the Counsellors had appointed the Marblehead committee was irrelevant, for Waterhouse had personally urged many of them to take this step.

As the battle continued, Waterhouse maintained that he had never denied the existence of the bonds, and that he had never received a farthing from them. With supporting evidence the Fellow retorted that Waterhouse most certainly had given the impression of denying taking bonds, that only now when proof was available did he for the first time admit it. Charge was met with countercharge, invective with invective, until in his final letter the Fellow mercilessly pilloried his adversary:

He talks of the dignity of moderation, who has exhausted our language of abusive terms; *he* talks of personality, who has loaded with opprobrious epithets a most respectable physician [Rand]; *he* declaims on the nicety of moral character, who has publicly violated the ninth commandment; *he* pretends to value himself for his "cardinal point of veracity," who before the world, has been proved guilty of repeated falshoods. . . . This gentleman has long been desirous of persuading the literati of *Europe*, that his transcendent talents have made him the object of envy and persecution in *America*. Regarded only with derision, even by the youngest Physicians in *Boston*, he was willing to relinquish his small claims to the friendship of his brethren, and invite the persecution, which was to lay the foundation for his greatness. . . . When W. accidentally was the first to receive vaccine matter from *Europe*, he thought it ought to be retained in his own possession; and this, not from any interested nature. . . . The vaccine fluid was, however, soon imported from *Europe* by others, and it was then rapidly diffused; . . . and other Physicians, as well as he, took the liberty to vaccinate. Then did he begin to hate his brethren of the faculty, and to store up instruments of vengeance. . . . The public was not long in discerning that W. knew no more of vaccination than others; and conceiving that, for what pains he had taken, he paid himself by praising his deeds in the newspapers, became averse from him, and the business of vaccinating was gradually transferred to the hands of more respectable Physicians, so that by the spring of 1806, his practice in *Boston* was nearly or quite annihilated. Then the direful passions, long pent up, began to rage with unconquerable fury; then the treasured weapons were drawn out, and some new *forged;* . . . disappointment and revenge were the causes which excited him to action. Let him now fly to the shades of retirement, that he may revolve in his mind new plots, and enjoy *those reflections* and *that reputation* to which the execution of former ones entitle him.[142]

To enhance his fame as "The Jenner of America," Waterhouse had started this fight. In the event he lost.[143]

VIII

Between 1799 and 1802 Waterhouse unquestionably contributed significantly to the diffusion of vaccination. While his friendship with Lettsom and Haygarth gave him an initial advantage, he worked hard to convince skeptics and to teach erring practitioners the importance of careful attention to the subject. He furnished active vaccine to Virginia and other Southern states through Thomas Jefferson, to New York through Valentine Seaman, and to many other communities. For nearly all this work he neither asked nor received any pay. From March, 1801, on, he maintained a continuity of cases and resupplied many who failed. He made himself through devotion to this cause one of the leading American vaccinators during the years when the practice was first becoming established.

At the same time, the basic discovery and the most important early works on vaccination were English. Waterhouse was not an originator, but a promoter. Nor was he the only American physician who imported the lymph. Dr. John Chichester successfully vaccinated one person in Charleston, South Carolina, in the winter of 1799 and subsequently tested him by variolation.[144] Dr. George Pearson sent a thread to David Hosack in New York late in 1798, but this and a second thread failed.[145] Dr. Edward Miller of New York received threads from Pearson in March, 1800, and in the following summer, also without success.[146] About the same time John Ring sent some virus to Dr. John Crawford of Baltimore, but he too was probably unable to propagate it.[147] Though these events played no part in actually establishing vaccination in the United States, they illustrate the obvious fact that Waterhouse was not the only physician sufficiently interested in the new procedure to try it out.

Moreover, several practitioners did successfully import vaccine. Thomas Manning of Ipswich received his shortly after Waterhouse, and the Massachusetts Medical Society obtained good virus in April, 1801. James Smith of Baltimore first vaccinated in that city on May 1, 1801, using lymph which had come from London. After testing his patient by variolation, he published the result and offered to dispense free vaccine to members of the profession. The following March he established the first vaccine institution in the United States.[148] Dr. John Redman Coxe introduced vaccination in Philadelphia on November 9, 1801, with virus received from Jefferson, but four or five days later equally good virus arrived from London.[149] Furthermore, even in Boston the newspapers printed a wealth of material promoting the practice which had not come from Waterhouse, and the nation's only professional journal, the *Medical Repository*, was fully alive to the importance of the new preventive.

Vaccination spread across the nation with remarkable rapidity. By the spring of 1802 it had reached all the major seaports and many smaller communities in the East, and as far west as Mississippi, Kentucky, and Ohio.[150] Though Waterhouse emphasized the difficulties he encountered and the people's reluctance to accept it, less ardent and contentious men viewed its rate of advance with equanimity. The editors of the *Medical Repository* believed by the summer of 1802 that "none of our readers at the present day can doubt that body of testimony on this subject which has been long since and repeatedly laid before the public."[151] Despite the opposition and prejudice which the discovery had encountered, they later observed, "We believe no improvement in the practice of physic, of any great importance, was ever adopted by the community with so much readiness as the vaccine inoculation." [152] Benjamin Russell, editor of the *Columbian Centinel* and a staunch advocate of the new practice, commented in December, 1802, that its progress had been "rapid and permanent." [153] For his part in this work, Waterhouse deserves much credit. Yet it is only reasonable to conclude that vaccination would have spread throughout the United States almost as quickly as it did had Waterhouse never lived.

In Boston, the physicians were evidently not as zealous or as vocal as Waterhouse in promoting this innovation. They probably did fail to continue vaccinating through the summer and fall of 1801.[154] Some may have at first questioned the value of the practice. Jackson in February, 1801, admitted to some loss of confidence in vaccination as a perfect security against smallpox. Yet it is certainly a travesty to declare or insinuate, as many writers beginning with Waterhouse have, that the profession as a whole hindered or opposed the introduction of vaccination. Aspinwall was the only doctor who publicly dissented, and his attitude was based at least in part on apparently honest doubts as to the ability of practitioners to be sure that they had communicated genuine cowpox to their patients.

The early interest, advocacy, and success of some physicians of Boston and nearby towns have already been described. To this may be added a statement made in 1808 by John Warren, Aaron Dexter, James Jackson, and John C. Warren:

> The high interest which this discovery excited in this country at the time of its annunciation, and the evidence, which was immediately offered by Dr. Jenner and his coadjutors, did, at a very early period, engage the attention of almost every individ-

ual among us in the medical profession; and that evidence was so perfectly satisfactory to the public, that a formal investigation of the subject by this [Massachusetts Medical] society, at that period, was altogether unnecessary.[155]

Though this statement, being late, has by itself little evidential value, Waterhouse himself wrote to Jefferson in June, 1801, that although the new practice had some adversaries even among the faculty, "The most eminent physicians in this region, as well as the most distinguished characters, in the two other learned professions, are advocates for this inoculation." In January, 1802, he wrote Valentine Seaman of New York that "all the old Physicians in Boston are advocates of the practice, & have introduced it into their own families;" the opposition came from "those who are candidates for fame, & business." Popular opinion, he continued, was also favorable.

While the common people see that characters the most distinguished for knowledge and rank in Society, as well as the most respectfull Physicians have their own children Inoculated & perceive that its opponents are the ignorant & the *interested*, they will duly appreciate the idle stories, here & there floating in the breath of rumour.[156]

In September, 1802, a group of twelve young physicians applied to the Board of Health for permission to use its office for a vaccine institution. Although they waited to announce the plan (which was fully approved by the "elders of the faculty") until after the health officials completed their experiment, this was certainly not because they needed to be themselves convinced.[157] Nor is it without significance that the American Academy of Arts and Sciences was the first organization in this country to honor Jenner formally, and that Harvard was the first university anywhere to confer upon him an honorary degree.[158]

If the physicians of Boston did not oppose vaccination, the possibility remains that they exhibited hostility toward Waterhouse personally. One of the Cambridge professor's principal targets in 1806 was Isaac Rand, but the latter produced several certificates testifying to his benevolent attitude during the critical period. Though this may not prove much, Waterhouse's own statement that he consulted Rand before publishing his attack on lay vaccinators in August, 1802, indicates that the two were not then inveterate enemies. And in 1807, apparently relieved by the previous year's act of catharsis, Waterhouse conceded that Rand was at an early period one of the most decided supporters of vaccination.[159] Waterhouse, it would seem, feeling that those who did not actively and vocally support him opposed him,[160] greatly magnified in his own mind the extent of his colleagues' aversion. He attributed to Rand and Warren, in connection with the Marblehead episode, a malicious attitude which there is no real evidence to believe they had. It is probable, moreover, that historians have tended to transfer back to an earlier period animosities engendered by Waterhouse's later difficulties with Harvard [161] and other subsequent controversies.

The existence of hostility toward Waterhouse is nevertheless evident. Samuel Brown, John C. Howard, and one or two other physicians attacked him in the newspapers. "Clericus" declared in the *Centinel* in 1803 that Waterhouse had "encountered prejudice and opposition at almost every step, and not the least from the faculty," while another writer noted that some people had termed his publications private advertisements.[162] An undercurrent of enmity is also apparent from the lack of articles by Boston physicians sympathetic to Waterhouse and from their failure to adopt his term, "kine pock."

Many writers have attributed this attitude in part to

political differences.[163] Waterhouse was not, like John Warren, a high Federalist. He did not look upon the election of Jefferson in 1800 as a national calamity: he reacted favorably to the conciliatory phrase, "We are all Republicans, we are all Federalists," in the President's Inaugural Address.[164] On the other hand he was not at this time an ardent Republican. Indeed, as late as the spring of 1806 a Boston magazine declared that Waterhouse paid "no regard to party politicks." [165] In the published correspondence between Waterhouse and John Adams, the first suggestion of political animus toward the Essex Junto—the extreme Federalist leaders of Massachusetts—does not occur until August, 1805. As late as December, 1809, two years after his son's break with the Federalists, Adams was apparently surprised to find that his friend had Republican leanings. "I did not before know," he wrote, "but you was one of those respectable People who do not read the *Patriot.*" It is from this letter that we learn of Waterhouse's "concern of Mind to write upon Politicks." [166] Writing to Lettsom on July 15, 1810, Waterhouse was even more explicit: "I was of this Fœderal party until within this year or two, as far as it regarded my voting; but I never was active or zealous; I, however, have abjured them since I find they prefer the honour of a foreign country to our own." [167]

Mild as these views were, Waterhouse's emphasis on Jefferson's support of vaccination and his failure to join the jihad against the President may not have endeared him to his Federalist colleagues.[168] It is clear, however, that politics had no significant connection with the introduction of vaccination. Waterhouse sent his first and most of his subsequent communications to the *Centinel*, one of the nation's most outspoken Federalist journals, and he transmitted his views to Connecticut in a letter to the high priest of Federalism, "Pope" Dwight of Yale. Samuel Brown's attempt to secure the virus in 1800 was denounced as an example of "*Jacobin benevolence*," and as another of the current weapons aimed "not only at law and property, but at civility, and the absolute rights of individuals!" [169] When the Republican *Independent Chronicle* in 1802 tried to make political capital out of Jefferson's support of vaccination and John Ring's opinion of "our illustrious President," Benjamin Russell, the editor of the *Centinel*, quickly replied that he considered Jefferson's patronage of the new preventive, long since acknowledged in his newspaper, "as amongst his most praise-worthy actions." And he added Ring's equally complimentary remarks about Adams.[170] Evidently Russell was unwilling to have anyone believe that Federalists supported vaccination less ardently than Republicans, and his own continued and vigorous promotion of the practice indicates that they were not.[171] Nor would the Massachusetts Medical Society, if actuated by political motives, have appointed William Eustis in 1806 to head a committee to investigate Waterhouse's charges. That Waterhouse was later an outspoken Republican is completely beside the point.

While it is difficult to perceive any correlation between political beliefs and attitudes toward vaccination, it is of course possible that Waterhouse's religious opinions [172] may have prejudiced others against him. It is equally true that petty jealousy evoked by his original appointment as Professor of Physic and by the recognition which he received from Jenner and others may have colored the views of some Bostonians. Nevertheless, Waterhouse's own actions and words solely in connection with the introduction of vaccination amply justified any existing hostility or distrust. He did not incur others' enmity because he inaugurated the practice, but because of the way he did it.

Throughout his newspaper articles and books Waterhouse exhibited a distinct tendency to self-glorification. He pointedly and unnecessarily emphasized his personal correspondence with Jenner and other British physicians.[173] He made great use of the first person singular pronoun. Repeatedly he pointed out that "I" first pronounced that cowpox would ever after secure a person from smallpox, that "I" warned against the dangers of spurious cases, that no patient "I" vaccinated had subsequently contracted smallpox, that "I" could not vouch for the practice of others.

Furthermore, Waterhouse studiously neglected the achievements of other physicians in this country. He disregarded almost completely American publications on vaccination, except for his own. Although the *Medical Repository* had previously printed an account of Jenner's work, cowpox, according to Waterhouse, was before his first article "a disease totally unknown, and till then unheard of in this quarter of the world." [174] The extensive literature submitted by others to the Boston newspapers and to the *Repository* received no credit in Waterhouse's *Prospect of Exterminating the Small Pox Part II, . . . a Narrative of Facts Concerning the Progress of the New Inoculation in America.*

Throughout this history Waterhouse conveyed the impression that he encountered little but opposition and stupidity. Almost invariably, he alluded to those who were vaccinating as early as 1800 only to discuss their failures or their requests to him for vaccine and instruction. It was remarkable, he wrote, that in neither New York, Philadelphia, Charleston, nor Savannah, did any of the vaccine repeatedly imported from England ever communicate the disease—despite Coxe's plain statement that he had successfully vaccinated with virus obtained from London.[175] Waterhouse noted in passing the failure of Baltimore doctors who used imported threads and declared that the physicians of Maryland, among others, were supplied from his stock through Jefferson.[176] He never mentioned James Smith. He referred to Manning's importation only once—in a newspaper article in December, 1800.[177] In his narrative Waterhouse described his June, 1801, request for reports of other practitioners' successfully tested cases of vaccination, but he failed to note the returns he received or any of the other public demonstrations of the efficacy of vaccination concluded in New England prior to the experiment supervised by the Boston Board of Health late in 1802.[178]

Waterhouse was equally reluctant to admit that the physicians of Boston had played a role in the introduction of vaccination. For example, he declared that in the summer of 1802 "The faculty in that town, with but one exception, had not given it their decided approbation and countenance." While it is not clear to which of the many supporters of vaccination Waterhouse referred, perhaps he had James Jackson in mind, for three pages later he mentioned Jackson's request to the Board of Health in 1801 for permission to test some of his patients by variolation. But Waterhouse immediately deflated whatever credit might have accrued to the young physician for this effort by calling him "my ingenious and esteemed pupil." One might suppose from this passage that Waterhouse had taught Jackson how to vaccinate.[179]

Waterhouse's account was not only incomplete, but in some cases lacking in candor. Particularly instructive is a careful examination of his treatment of the failures in November, 1800. At the time he attributed his own difficulties to a degeneration of the vaccine caused either by repeated human transfer or by cold weather. In April, 1801, however, after a letter from Jenner taught him the importance of taking the vaccine on the eighth or at the very latest the ninth day, Waterhouse acknowledged his error to Lettsom and Jenner and blamed his spurious cases on taking the lymph from the arms of his patients at too late a stage of the eruption.[180] In *Prospect Part II*, moreover, he in effect admitted that during the fall of 1800 he did not know when the vaccine should be taken.[181]

Yet earlier in this same volume, after referring to the warning against spurious cowpox in *Prospect* (Part I), Waterhouse wrote:

> I felt it my duty in November of the same year [1800] to acquaint the public, through the medium of the newspaper, that the kine-pock had, in many places, degenerated from its original mild character, and that this deviation appeared to have arisen from the inoculator taking his matter from the pustule at *too late a period*.[182]

Actually, the only suggestion in the newspaper publication to which Waterhouse was here referring (which first appeared not in November but on December 27) that taking the vaccine at too late a period caused spurious cases was a repetition of Jenner's warning, already printed in *Prospect* (Part I), against "matter taken from an ulcer in an *advanced stage*. . . ." [183] This caution, thrice given, was Waterhouse's only published statement prior to June, 1801, of the importance of taking the lymph at the proper time.[184] As his own experience proves, it was too indefinite to be of critical value.[185] No one, surely, would consider "an ulcer in an *advanced stage*" an accurate description of the vaccination pustule on, for example, the thirteenth day.

Waterhouse continued his narrative by relating that before Story's unfortunate mistake spread smallpox in Marblehead, Drury, who "took matter for his inoculations on the thirteenth day," [186]

had inoculated about forty persons, from the arm of his son whom I had vaccinated, but did not adhere to my directions respecting the *time* of taking the matter. ALL *that he inoculated took the small-pox, either casually, or by inoculation, one excepted.* . . . Although I saw clearly the cause of this disaster, (for I repaired immediately to Marblehead, and saw the chain of their calamity, and examined every link of it in conjunction with Dr. S. and Dr. D.) I found it vain to attempt to explain or palliate, but left its development to time, that infallible test of truth.[187]

Since Waterhouse himself was at this time taking vaccine too late, it seems more likely that Drury erred not so much because he failed to follow Waterhouse's directions —if Waterhouse gave him any—as because the directions were inadequate. A comparison of this account with Waterhouse's newspaper statements of November and December, 1800, moreover, reveals additional discrepancies. From these it appears that Waterhouse did go to Marblehead on November 12 or 13, when he obtained from Story a candid history of the introduction of the smallpox infection.[188] On December 20, however, Waterhouse wrote:

Having heard that several persons, who had been inoculated for the *Kine-Pox* at Marblehead, have since taken the small-pox, I wrote to the inoculator [Drury] in that town, requesting an acurate [*sic*] history of the business, and having waited a due time for an answer without receiving any, I can no longer defer giving you a few important facts respecting it. . . .

I inoculated . . . the son of a practitioner [Drury], a boy of about eight or nine years of age. His father brought him to my house in Cambridge. I put the thread in his arm, and gave his father a small portion of the same, but never saw nor heard any more of the boy afterwards, and of course I never knew whether he ever had the genuine *local affection*, and *specific fever*, which constitute that peculiar distemper, which I have said and still believe secures the human system from the small-pox. Yet from this boy's arm was taken, as I am informed, all the matter, with which all the others in Marblehead were inoculated. If the matter therefore, which I used, did not give the genuine disease in the *first* instance, which happens very frequently, then all the cases that followed it must of course be *spurious*, and absolutely incapable of securing the system from an attack of the small-pox. . . . The wide avenue which these facts open to uncertainty must be apparent to every discerning individual.[189]

In fact, as late as April, 1801, Waterhouse complained that he had been unable to obtain an accurate account of the accidents at Marblehead.[190] So much for his later claim that he immediately explored the circumstances with Drury and saw clearly the cause of his failure.

Were such inaccuracies Waterhouse's only sins, they might be overlooked, in view of his services, as the foibles of an egotistical and contentious character. But it is no longer possible to ignore his efforts to restrict the diffusion of vaccine in the late summer and early fall of 1800 in order to profit from a monopoly, or the bonds which he secured from other practitioners requiring them to remit one quarter of their profits in return for a supply of the virus. The existence of the bonds was known, or at least reported, as early as November, 1800. Publicly Waterhouse simply ignored that charge and John C. Howard's similar accusation in August, 1802. In letters to John C. Lettsom, Timothy Dwight, and Thomas Jefferson, however, he implied that the imputation was false, and Isaac Rand, John Warren, and Thomas Welsh all stated that in the fall of 1802 he had in effect denied taking such bonds.[191] Indeed, according to one member of the Massachusetts Medical Society, "Almost every physician in *Boston* is of opinion that

Dr. W. has on this subject used such expressions as to make them suppose he *did not take*, or meant to *deny taking* those bonds."[192]

In 1806, when Waterhouse could no longer evade the issue, he declared that the matter had been misrepresented, that he had never concealed the existence of the bonds, and that he had never intended to make any money from them. The following year he presented his full explanation. After the result of the test on his children in Aspinwall's hospital spread the fame of the new preventive, he wrote, he was deluged with "innumerable and embarrassing" requests for the virus.

By far the greatest number who applied for matter, and for instructions how to use it, were utter strangers to me. I discovered afterwards, that some of them were not even practitioners of physic, but *speculators in kine pock matter*. I saw what would be the consequence of this junction of avarice, ignorance and presumption, and warned the public in the *Centinel* against spurious matter.[193] The evil I predicted was spreading through the country, when I had a number of applicants of a different class from the first, namely, practitioners of known repute. After much consultation respecting the best mode of diffusing *genuine* vaccination, and repressing speculation in spurious matter, a plan of this sort was concluded on, and offered to me for consideration, viz. that I should supply these reputable physicians with matter continually, and with every instruction and assistance, even to visiting their district, if required; that they should notify to the public that I was at the head of their inoculation; and that they would in return give me a fourth part of the profits.[194] The gentlemen I refer to will doubtless do me the justice to declare that I objected to the last part of this agreement, remarking, that it was my duty as a professor, as well as my inclination, to diffuse all I know in medicine for the public good; but they absolutely refused to take matter from me on any other condition. They did not stop here;—they proposed that this scheme should be ratified by an exchange of bonds, while I thought a few lines expressive of each other's meaning would be sufficient;—they, however, urged that with bonds they could better regulate their own business with other practitioners; who were to be, as I found afterwards, subsidiary to them. I consented, but never relished the idea; so that this business of the *bonds* was a thing that did not originate with me; nor did I ever consider them of so much consequence as ever to ask any of these gentlemen to fulfil their conditions. . . . I never proposed to enrich myself by vaccination, and accordingly I never have. . . . [195]

It is entirely possible that Waterhouse's bonds failed to return much money. When he applied to the Massachusetts General Court in 1810 for some remuneration for his labors, a sympathetic committee reported that "although it is not pretended that he is poorer for what he has done in this new line of practice, yet your Committee are far from supposing that by means of it he has made himself rich." [196] No one, however, can carefully read the Waterhouse–Spalding–Bartlett letters without concluding that Waterhouse intended to profit from his original monopoly of the cowpox virus,[197] and that his later explanation of the bonds, so palpably improbable, was a complete fabrication. Though Waterhouse might well have charged a fee to cover his expenses and provide a reasonable income, his actions in the summer and early fall of 1800 were morally indefensible. They contradicted his own pretentions to philanthropy; they rendered his motives for warning against spurious cases suspect; and they fostered the spirit of commercialism which at first damaged the cause of vaccination. Furthermore, his later attempts to explain the bonds only served to convict him of lying. Knowing the basic facts, the physicians of Boston were fully justified in regarding Waterhouse with suspicion and hostility.

NOTES

I

1. See such standard works as J. H. Baas, *Outlines of the History of Medicine and the Medical Profession* (H. E. Handerson, trans., New York, 1889), 711; F. H. Garrison, *An Introduction to the History of Medicine* (4th ed., Philadelphia, 1929), 375; Arturo Castiglioni, *A History of Medicine* (E. B. Krumbhaar, trans., 2d ed., New York, 1947), 643; *Dictionary of American Biography* (Allen Johnson and Dumas Malone, eds., New York, 1928–36), XIX, 529-532; *Dictionary of American Medical Biography* (Howard A. Kelly and Walter L. Burrage, eds., New York, 1928), 1266-1269.

2. Thomas J. Pettigrew, *Memoirs of the Life and Writings of the Late John Coakley Lettsom* . . . (London, 1817), I, 121-122.

3. John Baron, *The Life of Edward Jenner, M.D., LL.D., F.R.S.* . . . (London, 1838), I, 385-389.

4. Edgar M. Crookshank, *History and Pathology of Vaccination* (Philadelphia, 1889), I, 425-429; "The Diffusion of Vaccination: History of Its Introduction into Various Countries," *British Medical Journal*, 1896, I, 1269; F. Dawtrey Drewitt, *The Life of Edward Jenner, M.D., F.R.S., Naturalist, and Discoverer of Vaccination* (London, 1931), 59; R. Hingston Fox, *Dr. John Fothergill and His Friends: Chapters in Eighteenth Century Life* (London, 1919), 375-376; James J. Abraham, *Lettsom: His Life, Times, Friends and Descendants* (London, 1933), 333-335, 363-364.

5. Josiah Bartlett, *A Dissertation on the Progress of Medical Science, in the Commonwealth of Massachusetts* (Boston, 1810), 28-29.

6. James Thacher, *American Medical Biography* . . . (Boston, 1828), I, 29.

7. "Death of Benjamin Waterhouse, M.D.," *Boston Medical and Surgical Journal*, XXXV (1846–47), 206. See also J. F. W. Lane, "Some Statistics of Small-Pox and Vaccination," *American Journal of the Medical Sciences*, n.s. XII (1846), 128.

8. O. W. Holmes, "The Medical Profession in Massachusetts," *Medical Essays 1842–1882* (The Writings of Oliver Wendell Holmes, Riverside Edition, IX, Boston, 1891), 349.

9. E. Warren, *The Life of John Warren, M.D.* . . . (Boston, 1874), 403-406; *The Life of John Collins Warren, M.D.* . . . (Boston, 1860), I, 77-78. See also E. Warren's intimation that Waterhouse was not "an authority that could be relied upon." *Ibid.*, I, 85.

10. S. D. Gross, *Lives of Eminent American Physicians and Surgeons of the Nineteenth Century* (Philadelphia, 1861). Gross credited David Hosack with being among the first, if not the very first, supporters of vaccination. *Ibid.*, 317.

11. E. H. Clarke and others, *A Century of American Medicine 1776–1876* (Philadelphia, 1876), 15.

12. H. A. Martin, "Jefferson as a Vaccinator," *North Carolina Medical*

Journal, VII (1881), 1-34. A Boston physician specializing in vaccination, Martin felt that the treatment he received from the ruling powers of the Massachusetts Medical Society was surpassed in scurrility only by that meted out to Waterhouse and Zabdiel Boylston.

13. S. A. Green, *History of Medicine in Massachusetts* . . . (Boston, 1881), 106-110.

14. Joseph Jones, *Contagious and Infectious Diseases, Measures for Their Prevention and Arrest* (Baton Rouge, 1884), 178-212; also in Jones, *Medical and Surgical Memoirs* . . . , III, part I (New Orleans, 1890), 310-344.

15. W. M. Welch, "The Jenner of America," Philadelphia County Medical Society, *Proceedings*, VII (1884–85), 172-201.

16. Wilson G. Smillie and others, "The Great Pioneers of Public Health in America 1610–1925," *American Journal of Public Health*, XLIII (1953), 1077-1084. The most important recent works on Waterhouse and vaccination are Robert H. Halsey, *How the President, Thomas Jefferson, and Doctor Benjamin Waterhouse Established Vaccination as a Public Health Procedure* (New York Academy of Medicine, History of Medicine Series, No. 5, New York, 1936); Reginald Fitz, " 'Something Curious in the Medical Line,' " *Bulletin of the History of Medicine*, XI (1942), 239-264; Josiah C. Trent, "Benjamin Waterhouse (1754–1846)," *Journal of the History of Medicine and Allied Sciences*, I (1946), 357-364. Other accounts include: J. H. Hunt, "Dr. Benjamin Waterhouse and the Introduction of Vaccination into the United States," *Brooklyn Medical Journal*, X (1896), 391-395; Francis R. Packard, *The History of Medicine in the United States* (Philadelphia, 1901), 91-92; *ibid.* (New York, 1931), I, 89-90; James G. Mumford, *A Narrative of Medicine in America* (Philadelphia, 1903), 276-277; Thomas F. Harrington, *The Harvard Medical School, a History, Narrative and Documentary 1782–1905* (New York, 1905), I, 91-93, 315-330; A. K. Stone, "Benjamin Waterhouse," *Boston Medical and Surgical Journal*, CLXXIV (1916), 285-286; George C. Whipple, *State Sanitation: a Review of the Work of the Massachusetts State Board of Health* (Cambridge, 1917), I, 10-14; J. W. Courtney, *Benjamin Waterhouse, M.D.: American Pioneer* (Communication faite au Vme Congrès International d'Histoire de la Médecine, Geneva, 1926), 3-7; Louis H. Roddis, *Edward Jenner and the Discovery of Smallpox Vaccination* (Menasha, 1930), 99-102; Henry R. Viets, *A Brief History of Medicine in Massachusetts* (Boston, 1930), 119-125; S. B. Woodward, "The Story of Smallpox in Massachusetts," *New England Journal of Medicine*, CCVI (1932), 1188-1190; C. J. Brim, "Benjamin Waterhouse (1754–1846): An Underestimated American Medical Pioneer," *Medical Life*, XLI (1934), 283-285; H. G. Partridge, "Benjamin Waterhouse," *Rhode Island Medical Journal*, XXIV (1941), 125-127; M. C. Leikind, "The Introduction of Vaccination into the United States," *Ciba Symposia*, III (1941–42), 1114-1124; Archibald Malloch, *Medical Interchange between the British Isles and America before 1801* (London, 1946), 43-44; Maurice B. Gordon, *Æsculapius Comes to the Colonies* . . . (Ventnor, N. J., 1949), 277-279; E. Ashworth Underwood, "Edward Jenner, Benjamin Waterhouse, and the Introduction of Vaccination into the United

States," *Nature*, CLXIII (1949), 823-828; I. B. Cohen, "Edward Jenner and Harvard University," *Harvard Library Bulletin*, III (1949), 352-357.

17. Edward Warren was obviously biased. Otherwise, Roddis (*op. cit.*, 102) remarked without amplification that Waterhouse was remembered for attempting to monopolize and commercialize vaccination. Courtney (*op. cit.*, 7) noted that Waterhouse was charged with commercializing the practice.

18. J. A. Spalding, *Dr. Lyman Spalding: the Originator of the United States Pharmacopœia* . . . (Boston, 1916), 52-109, *passim*.

19. M. C. Leikind, "An Episode in the History of Smallpox Vaccination in New Hampshire," *Bulletin of the History of Medicine*, VII (1939), 671-686.

20. Neither Halsey, Fitz, nor Trent appears to have used either Spalding's book or Leikind's article. Even Underwood, who did, declared (*loc. cit.*, 824, 825) that we must go to Waterhouse's own publications for a "true appreciation" of his difficulties, and that the letters published by Spalding and Leikind illustrated "an amusing incident, which was perhaps unavoidable in the social atmosphere of that time," but which was not representative of Waterhouse's character and work.

II

21. This was not the first publication on vaccination in the United States: see, "The Following Important Account of a New Publication in Great-Britain, by Dr. Jenner, Entitled *An Inquiry into the Causes and Effects of the Variolæ Vaccinæ, or Cow Pox*, Is Extracted from the *Analytical Review* for July, 1798," *Medical Repository*, II (1798–99), 255-258. This number appeared in December, 1798 (*ibid.*, 146). Despite Waterhouse's oft-quoted comment ("This publication shared the fate of most others on new discoveries. . . .") in *A Prospect of Exterminating the Small-Pox; Being the History of the Variolæ Vaccinæ, or Kine-Pox, Commonly Called the Cow-Pox; as It Has Appeared in England: with an Account of a Series of Inoculations Performed for the Kine-Pox, in Massachusetts* (Cambridge, 1800), 8 [hereafter cited as *Prospect* (Part I)], he wrote Lettsom on Apr. 10, 1799, that the news "excites the public curiosity as much as any thing that has occurred in the medical line since my remembrance." Thomas J. Pettigrew, "On the Priority of the Transmission of Cow-Pock Matter to America," *Philosophical Magazine and Journal* (London), XLIX (1817), 278. The *Centinel* article was also reprinted in *J. Russell's Gazette. Commercial and Political* (Boston), Mar. 21, 1799. When Waterhouse reprinted this account in *Prospect* (Part I), 4-8, he gave the date of its original publication as Mar. 12, an error which has frequently been repeated.

22. For the details of Waterhouse's work to this point, see Fitz, *loc. cit.*, 239-247.

23. Waterhouse, *Prospect* (Part I), 18-25; *Columbian Centinel*, July 19, Aug. 16, 1800; *Russell's Gazette*, Aug. 7, 1800. Waterhouse offered Aspinwall his choice of three patients for the first test, and he picked a

twelve-year-old servant boy, not one of Waterhouse's own children. The latter were tested shortly thereafter. Waterhouse, *Prospect* (Part I), 25; *Columbian Centinel*, Sept. 20, 1800.

24. *Ibid.*, Aug. 20, 1800.

25. Another term for cowpox, coined by Waterhouse.

26. Spalding, *op. cit.*, following p. 54.

27. The transcription published by Underwood, *loc. cit.*, 826, is somewhat more accurate than that in Spalding, *op. cit.*, 54.

28. *Ibid.*, 55-58.

29. *Ibid.*, 57-58; Leikind, *loc. cit.*, 682-683; *Columbian Centinel*, July 12, 16, Aug. 6, 1806; *The Repertory* (Boston), July 15, 1806. Waterhouse to Z. Bartlett, Oct. 1, 1800, MS. in New York Academy of Medicine. See Plate I. Waterhouse indicated in this letter that "I should much rather that all the physicians of your town would unite in the business, so as to cause the kine-pox to pervade your whole town," but sometime in October he also signed a note, "This certifies that I have given to Dr. Zacheus Bartlett the matter of the Kine-pox for the purpose of inoculation in Plymouth, but not to supply any other practitioner." See Plate II. Courtesy of Dr. William Finkelstein, of Waterbury, Connecticut. For David King, see C. F. Bartlett to Moses Brown, Newport, Nov. 11, 1800; for Dyer, see Brown to Bartlett, Providence, Oct. 17, 1800, Moses Brown Papers, Rhode Island Historical Society. With regard to King and Dyer, the direct evidence indicates only that they were restricted from giving the vaccine to anyone else. The presumption is that they paid, or promised to pay, a substantial fee to Waterhouse. I am indebted to Mr. Mack Thompson of the University of California at Riverside for calling the material in the Moses Brown Papers to my attention.

30. John Warren to John Collins Warren, Boston, Aug. 30, 1800, Warren Papers, IV, Massachusetts Historical Society. Halsey (*op. cit.* [note 16], 16) quoted this letter to illustrate his opinion that the profession in Boston so bitterly opposed anything emanating from Waterhouse that they would not even accept vaccine from him. No doubt Warren was slower than Waterhouse to see the prospective benefits of widespread vaccination: on July 8, 1800, he wrote his son that "The small pox will probably before long, go through this place. . . ." Warren Papers, IV.

31. Samuel Brown, *A Treatise on the Nature, Origin and Progress of the Yellow Fever* . . . (Boston, 1800), iii.

32. *Columbian Centinel*, Aug. 30, 1800.

33. *Ibid.*, Sept. 6, 1800. Halsey (*op. cit.*, 16) quoted the final portion of this letter (omitted here) as an example of the calumnious opposition endured by Waterhouse!

34. Spalding, *op. cit.*, 54-55. Note Waterhouse's implied assumption that Brown's motives were as selfish as his own. For Brown's temperate reply to Pedro, see *Columbian Centinel*, Sept. 10, 1800. The New Hampshire group, like Waterhouse, made their patients promise or even bond themselves not to allow anyone else to take lymph from their arms. The problem of preserving the monopoly against this threat is mentioned at some length in the letters printed by J. Spalding and Leikind. See especially, Leikind, *loc. cit.*, 684-685.

35. Spalding, *op. cit.*, 58. Spalding's identification of "Young Doctor Manning" as Samuel Manning of Cambridge is no doubt mistaken. It is not clear exactly when Manning first vaccinated. In 1829 he wrote, "by 2 spring ships from London in 1800 I rec'd from a brother Dr. I. C. Manning then in London persuing medical research vaccine virus direct from Dr. Woodvilles small pox vaccine institution . . . I communicated the disease . . . in the summer & autumn of 1800." Henry B. Shafer, *The American Medical Profession, 1783–1850* (Faculty of Political Science of Columbia University, ed., Studies in History, Economics and Public Law, No. 417, New York, 1936), 110. This claim being twenty-nine years late, it is possible to say only that Manning began vaccinating sometime before Sept. 24. By Oct. 3 he had already "inoculated many." *Annals of Medicine, for the Year 1800* (Edinburgh), V (1801), 479 (I have assumed that the letter here quoted, which is described only as dated from Ipswich, Massachusetts, was written by Manning).

36. James J. Putnam, *A Memoir of Dr. James Jackson* . . . (Boston, 1905), 218-222. Since Jackson has been derided as a follower of Woodville (in contrast to Waterhouse, the disciple of the unerring Jenner), it is worth pointing out that although Woodville blundered at first, he was well aware of it by the time Jackson studied with him. John C. McVail, "Cow-Pox and Small-Pox: Jenner, Woodville, and Pearson," *British Medical Journal*, 1896, I, 1271-1276. Moreover, Waterhouse himself frequently cited Woodville approvingly in his publications, and in April, 1801, he wrote to an English correspondent, "For more than a year I have held up these two eminent physicians [Jenner and Woodville] to the *American public*, as men who could scarcely err." Underwood, *loc. cit.* (note 16), 827.

37. Putnam, *op. cit.*, 221. Jackson admittedly hoped to "make a *mint* of money in a *bit* of time." But unlike Waterhouse, he made no great professions of philanthropy, nor did he attempt to keep others from the practice.

38. Spalding, *op. cit.*, 59.

39. Putnam, *op. cit.*, 222.

40. Columbian Centinel, Oct. 11, 1800.

41. John Warren to John Collins Warren, Boston, Oct. 11, 1800, Warren Papers, IV, Mass. Hist. Soc. Apparently Warren did not know of Jackson's ride to Ipswich.

42. John G. Coffin in *Columbian Centinel*, Oct. 15, 1800; Samuel Hunt, Jr., in *Boston Gazette. Commercial and Political*, Oct. 16, 1800. Jackson to Pickering, Nov. 13, 1800, Putnam, *op. cit.*, 223.

43. Spalding, *op. cit.*, 61-62; Leikind, *loc. cit.*, 680-681.

44. Levi to Josiah, Nov. 28, 1800, *ibid.*, 681.

45. Spalding, *op. cit.*, 64. Spalding had taught chemistry to medical students at Dartmouth.

46. *Ibid.*, 65. Emily A. Smith incorrectly credited Nathan Smith with practicing vaccination as early as August, 1800, on the basis of a letter to L. Spalding dated Aug. 25, 1800. *The Life and Letters of Nathan Smith, M.B., M.D.* (New Haven, 1914), 25. The full letter, dated (probably correctly) Aug. 25, 1801, is in Spalding, *op. cit.*, 89-90.

47. *Ibid.*, 66-67. See also, S. H. Rose to L. Spalding, Bridgehampton, N. Y., Nov. 17, 1800, *ibid.*, 67; N. Noyes to Spalding [Newburyport?], postmarked Oct. 14, 1800, *ibid.*, 73-74.

48. Edna F. Calder, ed., "Extracts from the Ames Diary," *Dedham Historical Register*, X (1899), 121. See also, the advertisements of Dr. Pickman in *The Salem Gazette*, Oct. 14, 1800, and of Dr. Torrey of Danvers, *ibid.*, Oct. 31, 1800.

49. C. F. Bartlett to Moses Brown, Sept. 5, Oct. 23, 28, 29, Nov. 11, Dec. 13, 22, 1800; Moses Brown to C. F. Bartlett, Oct. 17, 1800. Moses Brown Papers, R. I. Hist. Soc. See Plate III.

III

50. *Prospect* (Part I), 38-39. Waterhouse added a footnote, probably aimed at Samuel Brown: "Dr. W. is happy to find that every GENTLEMAN of the faculty in Boston and its vicinity, has understood this, and conducted accordingly." The pamphlet was advertised as "*This* day *published*," in the *Massachusetts Mercury* (Boston), Sept. 5, 1800.

51. Waterhouse, *Prospect* (Part I), 25-27. See Edward Jenner, *Further Observations on the Variolæ Vaccinæ, or Cow Pox* (London, 1799), 4.

52. Note that in form this was not a letter from Waterhouse to the paper.

53. *The Independent Chronicle: and the Universal Advertiser* (Boston), Oct. 30, 1800.

54. *Columbian Centinel*, Nov. 19, 1800 (reprinted in *Mass. Mercury*, Nov. 21, 1800); *Columbian Centinel*, Dec. 27, 1800 (reprinted in *Independent Chronicle*, Jan. 5, 1801).

55. For Waterhouse's descriptions, see, in addition to the newspapers cited above, *Independent Chronicle*, May 11, 1801; *Columbian Centinel*, Aug. 12, 1801; June 19, 1802; "Narrative of Facts Concerning the Inoculation of the Kine-Pock," *Medical Repository*, V (1801–02), 373-381; *A Prospect of Exterminating the Small Pox Part II, Being a Continuation of a Narrative of Facts Concerning the Progress of the New Inoculation in America; Together with Practical Observations on the Local Appearance, Symptoms, and Mode of Treating the Variola Vaccina, or Kine Pock . . .* (Cambridge, 1802), 8-9 (hereafter cited as *Prospect Part II*); Waterhouse to Valentine Seaman, Cambridge, Jan. 12, 1802, in Seaman, An Account of the Introduction of Vaccination or Kine-Pock Inoculation in N-York [New York, 1802?], 55-57, MS., New York Academy of Medicine.

56. *Independent Chronicle*, Nov. 16, 1801. See also, H. C. Bolton, "Memoir of Dr. Elisha North," Connecticut Medical Society, *Proceedings*, n.s. III, no. 4 (1887), 138-139; L. Bartlett to J. Bartlett, Kingston, Nov. 28, 1800, Leikind, *loc. cit.* (note 19), 681-682; *The Connecticut Courant* (Hartford), Jan. 25, 1802.

57. E. S. Bolton, ed., "Extracts from the Diary of James Parker of Shirley, Mass.," *New England Historical and Genealogical Register*, LXX (1916), 142. The persons mentioned in addition to the diarist were

apparently all his children except Eastman, who may have been a school teacher.

58. It is at least possible that Waterhouse demanded the usual *quid pro quo*, and that Story decided to use his own importation so that he would not feel obliged to send Waterhouse his cut.

59. *The Mercury and New-England Palladium* (Boston), Jan. 16, 1801 (hereafter cited as *New-England Palladium*). See also, *Columbian Centinel*, Nov. 19, Dec. 27, 1800; *Mass. Mercury*, Nov. 11, 1800; Waterhouse, *Prospect Part II*, 9-14; Mass. Hist. Soc., *Proceedings*, LII (1918–19), 322; Benjamin Lynde Oliver and William Currie, *Letters on the Kine Pox, and a Variety of Other Medical Subjects* (Philadelphia, 1802), 7. Additional interesting details may be found in *The Diary of William Bentley, D.D.* (Salem, 1905–14), II, 355-357.

60. Spalding, *op. cit.* (note 18), 58, 61. Waterhouse wrote Lettsom on Nov. 13, 1800, that the vaccine "fails in more than half I inoculate for several weeks past." Pettigrew, *loc. cit.* (note 21), 279.

61. *Columbian Centinel*, Nov. 19, 1800.

62. Waterhouse planned to inoculate a cow as soon as he received fresh vaccine from England (letter to Lettsom, Nov. 13, 1800, Pettigrew, *loc. cit.*, 279), and did in fact do so. He "obtained from her a crop of matter on the ninth day, which produced the disease in the human subject to perfection." Waterhouse to Jenner, Apr. 24, 1801, Baron, *op. cit.* (note 3), I, 441-442. No longer believing that repeated human transfer weakened the lymph, Waterhouse apparently did not repeat this experiment.

63. *Independent Chronicle*, Jan. 5, 1801 (reprinted from *Columbian Centinel*, Dec. 27, 1800). The promised communication never appeared. On Apr. 24, 1801, Waterhouse wrote to Jenner, "I here inclose a newspaper containing a communication written in the *clouds* last December. . . . When I had lost my way, and wandered into the wilds of conjecture, I stood still. I gave out that the winter was an unfavourable season for this new inoculation, and by that means I suspended the practice throughout the country from that period until the arrival of fresh matter and your letter." Baron, *op. cit.*, I, 440. In 1802 Waterhouse wrote of this period, "I perceived that the vaccine disease had deviated from its original character. . . . I endeavoured to account for this change . . . by persuading myself that the virus became milder as it receded from the cow; and that it would at length become effete by passing through a given number of human subjects." But the experience of Marblehead and the writings of certain English physicians had led some to believe that cowpox increased in virulence with time. Waterhouse continued: "I silently entertained another whim, that the cold weather aggravated this disease. . . . I wrote to . . . England for a fresh supply of the vaccine virus, and gave out that the present season was less favourable to the inoculation than the spring." *Prospect Part II*, 14-15. See also, Fitz, *loc. cit.* (note 16), 251. The reiterated statement that he "gave out" that the winter was unfavorable may have been a reference to the letters published in the *Columbian Centinel* on Aug. 20 and Nov. 19 (the Dec. 20 letter did not mention weather), but more probably referred to personal communications with those who requested vaccine or vaccination. On Nov. 22, 1800, for example,

Waterhouse wrote Moses Brown, "Respecting the supplying Dr. Bartlett with the matter of the kine-pox, I shall return him the same answer I have uniformly given to all applicants for a week or two past, namely that I decline diffusing any more matter untill the opening of the Spring, being firmly persuaded that the winter season is not the most favourable for conveying the infection and conducting the disease to the greatest advantage." Waterhouse also pointed out that "Without the greatest care & attention the matter depreciates & becomes spurious. It has done so with every practitioner [torn] and has I fear degenerated in the hands of many of those whom I have supplied." He did not mention his own difficulties. Moses Brown Papers, R. I. Hist. Soc. The phrase "gave out," and this letter, suggest that Waterhouse used the cold-weather theory chiefly as an excuse; his public letters stressed the idea that repeated human transfer caused the vaccine to deteriorate. Apparently Waterhouse actually believed that both theories offered possible explanations for his failures. Letters to Lettsom, Nov. 13, 1800, and Dec. 13, 1800, Pettigrew, *loc. cit.*, 279-280. Waterhouse did not until some time later explicitly and publicly admit his failure to keep the virus going: one might assume from the Dec. 20 letter that despite his difficulties he was still attempting to vaccinate.

64. Waterhouse to Spalding, Dec. 18, 1800, Spalding, *op. cit.*, 60. Waterhouse did publish a letter from James Mann reporting his successful vaccinations (*Columbian Centinel*, Jan. 14, 1801); and an answer (*Independent Chronicle*, Mar. 16, 1801) to an advertisement (*ibid.*, Jan. 26, 1801) of an alleged case of the failure of cowpox to protect against smallpox.

IV

65. *Annals of Medicine, for the Year 1800* (Edinburgh), V (1801), 479; Joseph B. Felt, *History of Ipswich, Essex, and Hamilton* (Cambridge, 1834), 197; Shafer, *op. cit.* (note 35), 110; letter from an Essex County physician (undoubtedly Manning) to Jackson, *Columbian Centinel*, Apr. 8, 1801. Manning also made a similar test in May, 1801. Massachusetts law prohibited variolation in any town without the voters' permission in town meeting.

66. Boston Board of Health, "Report [on Vaccination Experiment]" (Broadside, Boston, Dec. 16, 1802), reproduced in *New England Journal of Medicine*, CCXVII (1937), 534.

67. *Columbian Centinel*, Feb. 14, 1801. In a temperate and reasoned letter supporting vaccination an anonymous writer pointed out in *The Salem Gazette*, Dec. 30, 1800, that although some trials had failed, "nine Physicians out of ten in this country, and probably a much larger proportion in Europe, who have subjected their patients to the test, have been successful."

68. *Columbian Centinel*, Jan. 14, 1801.

69. *Ibid.*, July 16, 1806.

70. *Independent Chronicle*, Jan. 5, 1801. For another successful test, probably in Rhode Island, of a girl vaccinated in December, 1800, see

Dorcas Earl to Moses Brown, Apr. 30, 1801, Moses Brown Papers, R. I. Hist. Soc.

71. *Independent Chronicle*, Jan. 5, 1801. The author was identified as "B****," which suggests that he may have been Samuel Brown.

72. *Columbian Centinel*, Jan. 14, 1801. For contemporary strictures on Waterhouse's first pamphlet by a competent and sympathetic critic who was not involved in the local situation, see John Ring, *A Treatise on the Cow-Pox* . . . (London, 1801–03), I, 443-459.

73. *Columbian Centinel*, Feb. 14, 1801. Wheelock had a fairly severe local reaction at the site of inoculation and some constitutional symptoms. While he may possibly have been infected with the smallpox virus, he had only one real pock and his affliction was much milder than usual for inoculated smallpox. Almost certainly his vaccination had afforded him a large degree of, if not perfect, protection. It is of course true that vaccination is not a perfect preventive of smallpox.

74. *Columbian Centinel*, Feb. 25, 1801.

75. *Ibid.*, Mar. 14, 1801.

76. *Ibid.*, Apr. 8, 1801. The author (identified only as a physician of Essex County, but undoubtedly Manning) also pointed out that occasionally individuals had smallpox more than once, and suggested that this might happen with cowpox. Jackson still believed that Wheelock's case represented a deviation from the rule, but he also wrote, "No man is less ready than I am to deny the power attributed to cow pox, as generally existing." Waterhouse also refused to admit that Wheelock had smallpox. *Ibid.*, Apr. 1, 1801. Jackson's second letter and a portion of the first were reprinted in Putnam, *op. cit.* (note 36), 230-233.

V

77. Their cooperation has been amply described by Halsey, *op. cit.* (note 16).

78. *New-England Palladium*, May 1, 26, 1801.

79. *Columbian Centinel*, Apr. 8, 1801.

80. Actually one case was successful. *Ibid.*, June 18, 1806.

81. Waterhouse to Rand, Apr. 5, 1801, *ibid.*, July 2, 1806. The emphatic type of the printed letter, which was not all in the original, has been omitted.

82. See Waterhouse to Lettsom, Apr. 6, 1801, Pettigrew, *op. cit.* (note 2), III, 212; to an unknown English correspondent, Apr. 14, 1801, Underwood, *loc. cit.* (note 16), 827.

83. *Columbian Centinel*, June 18, July 12, 16, 1806.

84. It is significant that Waterhouse pressed this request much more assiduously than his offer to place himself under the "advice and direction" of the Society.

85. The pertinent extracts from the records of the Society are in Walter L. Burrage, *A History of the Massachusetts Medical Society . . . 1781–1922* (Norwood, Mass., 1923), 58-59. The letters were from Elisha Story,

Thomas Manning, John D. Treadwell of Salem, and Waterhouse. See also, *Columbian Centinel*, July 16, 23, 30, Aug. 2, 1806.

86. *Ibid.*, June 27, 1801. The notice was reprinted in *Independent Chronicle*, July 2, 1801; *Conn. Courant*, July 13, 1801; *The Spectator* (New York), July 4, 1801 (Halsey, *op. cit.*, 29-30); and no doubt in other newspapers. It is worth noting that this inquiry was far from scientific: Waterhouse asked for favorable reports only.

87. Valentine Seaman, "A Report on the Vaccine or Kine-Pox Inoculation in New-York," *Medical Repository*, V (1801–02), 236-238. Jackson had sent virus to New York in the fall of 1800, but it had proved spurious on trial. David Hosack to John Redman Coxe, Jan. 15, 1802, Coxe, *Practical Observations on Vaccination: or Inoculation for the Cow-Pock* (Philadelphia, 1802), 128-129. Seaman claimed to have received on May 22, 1801, the first genuine vaccine to reach New York, but some from Elisha North of Goshen, Conn., may have preceded it. Seaman, *op. cit.* (note 55), 8; Bolton, *loc. cit.* (note 56), 140-142.

88. Waterhouse to Jenner, Apr. 8, 1802, Baron, *op. cit.* (note 3), I, 593-594; W. R. LeFanu, *A Bio-Bibliography of Edward Jenner 1749–1823* (Philadelphia, [1951]), 60-62. The instructions are reproduced in *ibid.*, plate XVIII.

89. *Columbian Centinel*, July 15, Aug. 5, 12, Oct. 7, Nov. 7, Dec. 16, 1801; June 19, July 17, 28, Nov. 13, 1802; *Independent Chronicle*, June 18, 1801; June 28, July 15, Aug. 5, 1802; *New-England Palladium*, July 21, 1801; Jan. 19, Mar. 2, Apr. 16, May 21, 1802.

90. *Ibid.*, May 29, June 2, 1801. It is, however, quite possible that the anonymous physician was in this case Waterhouse; the argumentative style and some of the phrases suggest as much. If so, it is particularly significant that the writer suggested that "A Tradesman" could obtain from the eldest physician in the North End "a chain of information" which would convince him of the value of vaccination.

91. *Independent Chronicle*, Nov. 16, 1801.

92. *New-England Palladium*, July 17, 1801. The vaccinator was Dr. Benjamin Page, Jr.

93. *Ibid.*, Aug. 14, 21, 1801. For further details, see Spalding, *op. cit.* (note 18), 88. L. Spalding made a second public test in July, 1802. *Ibid.*, 104-105; *Columbian Centinel*, July 17, 1802.

94. *New-England Palladium*, Oct. 23, 1801; *Independent Chronicle*, Oct. 29, 1801. By March, 1802, Cooley claimed to have vaccinated more than 600 persons, a large number of whom had been tested both by inoculation and exposure to patients. *Conn. Courant*, Mar. 1, 1802. He was evidently much interested in the subject: one of the curiosa of vaccination is an edition of Jenner's *Inquiry* reprinted from the second London edition for Cooley in Springfield, Mass., in 1802. See also, *Conn. Courant*, Oct. 19, 1801.

95. *Independent Chronicle*, Nov. 9, 1801.

96. *New-England Palladium*, Feb. 23, June 1, 1802.

97. *Columbian Centinel*, Aug. 7, 1802.

98. *Ibid.*, July 11, Sept. 26, 1801; *New-England Palladium*, July 7, 1801; Feb. 26, 1802; *Independent Chronicle*, May 20, 1802.

99. *Columbian Centinel*, May 19, June 12, Sept. 18, 1802; *New-England Palladium*, July 31, 1801; Mar. 12, May 18, 21, July 16, 1802; *Independent Chronicle*, Aug. 24, 1801; Mar. 11, June 7, July 19, 1802.

100. *New-England Palladium*, June 30, July 24, 1801; *Columbian Centinel*, July 24, 1802.

101. The continued skepticism of some Bostonians may be documented by the continued existence of Aspinwall's inoculation hospital. See especially his advertisement, *Independent Chronicle*, June 21, 1802. Since the newspapers rarely published anything derogatory to vaccination, the arguments of the opposition must in general be inferred from those used by Waterhouse and others to combat it.

102. Benjamin Waterhouse, "Small Pox and Kine Pock," *Boston Medical Intelligencer*, IV (1826–27), 33.

103. *Columbian Centinel*, Sept. 20, 1800.

104. *Independent Chronicle*, Oct. 1, 1801. The advertisement was repeated in *ibid.*, Oct. 8, 15, 22, 29, 1801.

105. *Ibid.*, Oct. 5, 1801.

106. *New-England Palladium*, Oct. 13, 1801.

107. *Independent Chronicle*, Oct. 15, 1801.

108. Walter C. Alvarez, "Some Correspondence Relating to the Introduction of Vaccination into America," *California and Western Medicine*, XXIII (1925), 584. Aspinwall, so far as I know, wrote nothing publicly about any time limitation on the efficacy of cowpox, but he may have made such statements orally or in private letters.

109. *Independent Chronicle*, Nov. 2, 1801.

110. *Ibid.*, Oct. 29, 1801. For a similar argument elsewhere, see *Conn. Courant*, Mar. 1, 1802. In December, 1801, Dr. B. L. Oliver wrote that although the physicians of Salem had confidence in cowpox, it was "generally thought" that they did not yet possess "all the diagnostic signs, necessary for ascertaining when the system is secured from the small-pox by the vaccine disease." He expected that time would soon remove the obscurity. Oliver and Currie, *op. cit.* (note 59), 8-9.

111. *Independent Chronicle*, Nov. 9, 1801.

112. Alvarez, *loc. cit.*, 584.

113. *Columbian Centinel*, Apr. 1, 1801; Boston Board of Health, Records (1799–1806), 132, 154-157, 159-160, 164, 167, MS. in Boston Public Library.

114. *Columbian Centinel*, May 19, 22, 1802; Aspinwall's advertisement, *Independent Chronicle*, June 21, 1802; Waterhouse, *Prospect Part II*, 49. Not having been through a general smallpox inoculation since 1792, Boston undoubtedly contained thousands of susceptible inhabitants.

115. Boston Board of Health, "Report," *New England Journal of Medicine*, CCXVII (1937), 534; Waterhouse, *Prospect Part II*, 51.

116. Boston Board of Health, *loc. cit.*; *idem*, Records (1799–1806), 215-222, 225-229; Boston Registry Department, *Records Relating to the Early History of Boston* (Boston, 1900–09), XXXV, 133-134; *Columbian Centinel*, July 3, 24, Aug. 18, 25, Dec. 18, 1802; *New-England Palladium*, June 25, July 2, Aug. 20, 27, Dec. 21, 1802; *Independent Chronicle*, July 1, Dec. 20, 1802; Spalding, *op. cit.*, 107-109. The test was delayed

until November because of difficulties in securing the smallpox virus. Even Aspinwall had none that was good at this time. Though the experiment has often been described, no one, I believe, has noted that two members of the Board of Health, Ozias Goodwin and Daniel Scott, offered their own sons for the test.

117. *Prospect Part II*, 64.

VI

118. Pettigrew, *op. cit.* (note 2), III, 212. This suggests that rumors about Waterhouse's effort to monopolize the practice had reached England.

119. *Independent Chronicle*, May 11, 1801, reprinted from *Connecticut Journal* (New Haven), Apr. 29, 1801. The letter has been reprinted in Halsey, *op. cit.* (note 16), 24-27.

120. *Ibid.*, 42-43. Waterhouse did not explicitly deny in this letter that he accepted and approved (if he did not initiate) the offer of one quarter of the profits, but he certainly gave that impression. Ironically, Halsey pointed out (p. 3) Jefferson's antipathy to making money from a monopoly. Thoroughly imbued with Waterhouse's side of the story, but apparently knowing nothing about the bonds or the Waterhouse–Spalding letters, Halsey concluded (p. 57) that Waterhouse had no desire to restrict the use of vaccination and made every effort to spread the knowledge of its value. "Though offered large financial inducements for exclusive rights he refused them as a 'vile conspiracy' and took every adequate means to prevent the organization of monopolies in various states and towns." See also, Fitz, *loc. cit.* (note 16), 248. More recently, Laurence Farmer has noted that this letter reflected sadly on the other physicians' (but not Waterhouse's) ethical standards. *Doctors' Legacy: a Selection of Physicians' Letters 1721–1954* (New York, 1955), 78.

121. *Columbian Centinel*, Aug. 13, 1806. A MS. copy of the letter in the Harvard Medical School Library varies from the printed version in minor ways.

122. Waterhouse to L. Spalding, Sept. 25, 1800, Spalding, *op. cit.*, 58.

123. *Columbian Centinel*, July 28, 1802. Also printed in *Independent Chronicle*, Aug. 5, 1802 (without the final section beginning, "I should not have glanced . . ."); and in Waterhouse, *Prospect Part II*, 40-48.

124. *Ibid.*, 48.

125. *Columbian Centinel*, July 31, 1802. After Waterhouse's letter appeared on July 28, Howard first wrote for an explanation or apology. Receiving no answer, he then requested a friend, William Sullivan, to call upon the Cambridge physician. Taking his brother as a witness, Sullivan went to Waterhouse, who, after some discussion, reluctantly drew up this notice, which the Sullivans deemed acceptable. They handed it to Howard, who, presumably, inserted it in the newspaper. *Ibid.*, Dec. 30, 1807.

126. *Ibid.*, Aug. 11, 1802.

127. Howard later signed the physicians' statement for the December, 1802, report on vaccination by the Board of Health, and he was one of the young physicians who established a vaccine institution in Boston immediately following the publication of this report. *Independent Chronicle*,

Dec. 23, 1802. Shortly thereafter, he resumed general practice. *Columbian Centinel*, Mar. 9, 1803. He was admitted to the Massachusetts Medical Society in 1803. Walter L. Burrage, *The Massachusetts Medical Society: a Catalogue of the Honorary and Past and Present Fellows 1781–1931* (Boston, 1931), 124.

128. *Columbian Centinel*, Aug. 14, 1802.

129. In *Prospect Part II*, 48-49, Waterhouse said that he deemed it his duty to attack the practice of vaccination by mechanics and day laborers but that before sending the letter published on Aug. 11, he read it to the president of the Massachusetts Medical Society (Isaac Rand), "determining to suppress it, should the principles and design of it, meet his disapprobation. Its publication, notwithstanding, let loose all '*the angry passions*.'" As an example he cited, but did not quote, Howard's reply.

130. *Columbian Centinel*, July 12, 1806. This is Rand's version of the conversation. Waterhouse declared that Rand was perverting the facts (*ibid.*, July 16, 1806), but John Warren, Thomas Welsh, and others supported Rand in substance (*ibid.*, July 19, Aug. 6, 1806).

131. Though dated 1802 on the title page, it actually appeared about Feb. 1, 1803. See William Hilliard's advertisement, *Columbian Centinel*, Feb. 5, 1803.

132. *Ibid.*, Mar. 30, Apr. 9, May 21, June 15, 25, July 16, Nov. 26, 1803; Apr. 11, May 26, Nov. 7, 28, Dec. 1, 1804; May 4, 1805.

VII

133. *Columbian Centinel*, Apr. 19, 23, 1806. A third letter (*ibid.*, May 31, 1806) was devoted to technical matters that had nothing to do with Waterhouse's controversy with the Society.

134. *Dict. Amer. Biog.*, VI, 193-194.

135. This description of the letter was by the Society's chief defender. *Columbian Centinel*, July 12, 1806.

136. *Ibid.*, Aug. 2, 1806. Quoting the letter from memory, Waterhouse wrote that it was "meant to convey nothing disrespectful."

137. *Ibid.*, June 18, July 9, 12, 16, 19, 1806.

138. *Ibid.*, June 18, 1806.

139. *Ibid.*, July 2, 1806.

140. Warren Papers, VI, Mass. Hist. Soc.

141. *Columbian Centinel*, July 9, 1806.

142. *Ibid.*, July 30, 1806.

143. For the full record of this extended controversy, see *ibid.*, Apr. 19, 23, June 18, 21, July 2-Aug. 13, Aug. 23, 1806. *Repertory*, July 15, 1806. Two or three years prior to this controversy, Waterhouse had gone to the Society seeking the letter to Rand. Unable to find it in the files, Waterhouse turned to Rand himself. The latter still had it and gave it back to Waterhouse at his request. In September, 1806, after the newspaper battle was over, Waterhouse "returned" the letter to the Massachusetts Medical Society to be placed on its files where it belonged, remarking that "had it not been over looked & forgotten, . . . it would have been returned as

it indeed ought, directly on my taking a copy of it." Copies of letters to John Warren and to the President and Council of the Massachusetts Medical Society, both dated Cambridge, Sept. 28, 1806, in Harvard Medical School Library. The effrontery of this man was monumental. Two or three years prior to this episode, Jackson, J. C. Warren, and a few other young physicians organized a private medical improvement society which met weekly. In 1806 they published a series of unsigned articles on vaccination in the *Repertory*, several of which contained allusions obviously directed against Waterhouse. The most pointed was one by Warren ridiculing the term "kine pox" in the issue of Sept. 2. For the whole series, see *ibid.*, June 3, 24, July 11, 22, Aug. 5, 22, Sept. 2, 26, 30, Oct. 14, 28, Nov. 11, Dec. 9, 1806. See also, E. Warren, *Life of J. C. Warren*, I, 77-78; Putnam, *op. cit.* (note 36), 252-253.

VIII

144. Chichester received his vaccine from Pearson and tried it on several persons, but on only one did it take. His reason for going no further does not appear. Nathaniel H. Rhodes, "Evidence of the Precise Date of the Cow-Pock in America," *Philosophical Magazine* (London), XVI (1803), 252-253. Chichester's claim was noted by Fox, *op. cit.* (note 4), 376n.

145. Hosack to J. R. Coxe, New York, Jan. 15, 1802, Coxe, *op. cit.* (note 87), 128; Thacher, *op. cit.* (note 6), 28n. See also, Oliver and Currie, *op. cit.* (note 59), 11-12.

146. *Medical Repository*, III (1799–1800), 310; *ibid.*, IV (1800–01), 79; *Mass. Mercury*, Apr. 8, 1800.

147. Ring, *op. cit.* (note 72), I, 459. See also, J. R. Quinan, "The Introduction of Inoculation and Vaccination into Maryland, Historically Considered," *Maryland Medical Journal*, X (1883–84), 118; J. E. Wilson, "An Early Baltimore Physician and His Medical Library," *Annals of Medical History*, ser. 3, IV (1942), 66.

148. Quinan, *loc. cit.*, 118-119, 129-131; Whitfield J. Bell, Jr., "Dr. James Smith and the Public Encouragement for Vaccination for Smallpox," *Annals of Medical History*, ser. 3, II (1940), 502-504; H. C. Brooke, "A Proposal for a Free Vaccine Clinic in Baltimore in 1802," *Bulletin of the Institute of the History of Medicine*, III (1935), 83-91.

149. Coxe, *op. cit.*, 120-122. In the fall of 1801 Dr. Samuel Cooley of Bolton, Mass., noted that his vaccine "came to me with Dr. Jenner's treatise," which suggests that he too may have imported it directly from England. *Conn. Courant*, Oct. 19, 1801. See also, *ibid.*, Jan. 25, 1802.

150. Coxe, *op. cit.*, 130-134, 151-152; John Spence, "Observations on the Inoculation of the Kine-Pock," *Medical Repository*, V (1801–02), 381-387; *Columbian Centinel*, June 19, 1802; Madge E. Pickard and R. Carlyle Buley, *The Midwest Pioneer, His Ills, Cures, & Doctors* (Crawfordsville, Ind., 1945), 23.

151. Review of Coxe, *op. cit.*, in *Medical Repository*, VI (1802–03), 206.

152. Review of Waterhouse, *Prospect Part II*, in *Medical Repository*, VI (1802–03), 410.

153. *Columbian Centinel*, Dec. 18, 1802.

154. Waterhouse to Matthias Spalding, Oct. 20, 1801, Alvarez, *loc. cit.* (note 108), 584; *Columbian Centinel*, Dec. 16, 1801. An anonymous Boston physician, whose MS. "Kine pox inoculation records" are in the Boston Medical Library, vaccinated Oct.-Nov. 1800, Apr.-June 1801, and Mar.-June 1802.

155. "Report on Vaccination," Mass. Med. Soc., *Medical Communications*, vol. I, no. 2, part 2 (1808), 90.

156. *Prospect Part II*, 29; Waterhouse to Seaman, Cambridge, Jan. 12, 1802, in Seaman, *op. cit.* (note 55), 44-45.

157. Boston Board of Health, Records (1799–1806), 224, MS. in Boston Public Library; *Columbian Centinel*, Dec. 22, 1802; *Independent Chronicle*, Dec. 23, 1802; *New-England Palladium*, Dec. 24, 1802. The members of the institution were John Fleet, Jr., William Ingalls, Samuel Brown, Thomas Danforth, John G. Coffin, James Jackson, Benjamin Shurtleff, Jacob Gates, Isaac Rand, 3d, Samuel Hunt, Jr., John C. Warren, and John C. Howard. See also, the decisive statement published by the Boston Dispensary, *Columbian Centinel*, June 25, 1803.

158. Baron, *op. cit.* (note 3), II, 449-451; I. B. Cohen, "Edward Jenner and Harvard University," *Harvard Library Bulletin*, III (1949), 347-358. In Philadelphia, on the other hand, when Jenner was proposed as an associate of the College of Physicians, he failed of election. S. Weir Mitchell, *Celebration of the Centennial Anniversary of the Institution of the College of Physicians of Philadelphia* [Philadelphia, 1887], 32.

159. *Columbian Centinel*, July 19, 30, 1806; Dec. 12, 1807; *Prospect Part II*, 48-49.

160. Urging L. Spalding to take a partnership with Cutter, Waterhouse remarked in a letter dated Sept. 15, 1800, "*Besides*, 'he that is not with you' as the Bible says '*will be against you*.'" Spalding, *op. cit.* (note 18), 56.

161. William Coolidge Lane, "Dr. Benjamin Waterhouse and Harvard University," Cambridge Historical Society, *Publications*, IV (1909), 5-22; I. B. Cohen, *Some Early Tools of American Science* (Cambridge, 1950), 103-106; Samuel Eliot Morison, *Three Centuries of Harvard 1636–1936* (Cambridge, 1936), 222-223.

162. *Columbian Centinel*, May 21, June 15, 1803. These writers may well have been influenced by Waterhouse's recently published *Prospect Part II*.

163. The most vigorous expression of this theory is in C. J. Brim, "Benjamin Waterhouse (1754–1846): An Underestimated American Medical Pioneer," *Medical Life*, XLI (1934), 277-301. Displaying a remarkable inattention to the significance of dates and changing opinions, Brim, who cited no sources, blundered badly. For example, he quoted (p. 284) as one letter from John Adams to Waterhouse dated Sept. 10, 1800, parts of two letters, one with the date given, the other actually dated Dec. 18, 1809. For the original letters, see John Adams, *Statesman and Friend: Correspondence of John Adams with Benjamin Waterhouse 1784–1822*

(Worthington C. Ford, ed., Boston, 1927), 10-11, 45-46. Brim's findings are obviously worthless.

164. For a contemporary expression of Waterhouse's political views, see his letter to an unknown English correspondent, dated Apr. 14, 1801, in Underwood, *loc. cit.* (note 16), 827. In a letter to M. Spalding dated Apr. 15, 1802, Waterhouse noted, "[Caleb Strong] has a majority of votes over [Elbridge] Gerry of *ten thousand.*" Alvarez, *loc. cit.*, 584. Unfortunately Waterhouse neglected to indicate whether this result pleased or dismayed him. Incomplete election returns in the *Columbian Centinel* of Apr. 14, 1802, showed Strong (transcribed "Geo. Stroud" by Alvarez), the Federalist candidate for governor, leading Gerry, the Republican, by a vote of 23,577 to 14,893.

165. "Sketch of the Life of Benjamin Waterhouse, M.D." *The Polyanthos,* II (1806), 85-86.

166. Adams, *op. cit.*, 28-29, 45. But see Adams to Waterhouse, Jan. 3, 1806, just after the election of Fisher Ames, a leading Essex-Junto Federalist, as president of Harvard (he declined): "I wish you may have all the Satisfaction in him [Ames] which you anticipate and I have no reason to doubt that you will." *Ibid.*, 33. Actually Adams was none too happy about the choice. The *Boston Patriot* was a leading Republican newspaper.

167. Pettigrew, *op. cit.* (note 2), II, 490.

168. Waterhouse later claimed that this was the case, in a letter to Dr. James Tilton dated Cambridge, Mar. 24, 1815, copy in Harvard Medical School Library. However, Waterhouse wrote this letter, which related his past and present political services and sufferings in the cause of Republicanism, in the hope of obtaining a government job and may well have dressed the story up.

169. *Columbian Centinel*, Sept. 6, 1800. "Jacobin" was of course a favorite Federalist epithet for Jeffersonians. Incidentally, William Aspinwall was active in Republican party politics.

170. *Independent Chronicle*, Nov. 11, 1802; *Columbian Centinel*, Nov. 20, 1802. The *New-England Palladium*, another Federalist paper, had earlier remarked (Feb. 26, 1802), "President JEFFERSON may be considered as the great patron of the Kine-Pock inoculation in *America*."

171. The selectmen of Milton, in a well-deserved tribute, addressed Russell in 1809 as "the Man whose exertions have been so ably engaged from the earliest period to make evident that great blessing, and who has uninteruptedly [*sic*] persevered in that benevolent pursuit." *Columbian Centinel*, Nov. 22, 1809. For a brief account of the circumstances, see Green, *op. cit.* (note 13), 110-111.

172. Raised a Friend, Waterhouse retained his sympathy for this sect, but apparently was not actually a member of the Society. His daughter married a Unitarian minister, son of Harvard's professor of divinity.

173. See, for example, J. B. Blake, "An Unrecorded Jenner Imprint," *Journal of the History of Medicine and Allied Sciences*, IX (1954). 233-234. S. E. Morison has remarked that after receiving the snuffbox from Jenner, Waterhouse became "insufferably vain." *New England Journal of Medicine*, CCXVI (1937), 82.

174. *Prospect Part II*, 77. See above, note 21. Seaman gave the Med-

ical Repository full credit for its early and continuing work in publicizing vaccination. *Op. cit.* (note 55), 3-6.

175. *Prospect Part II*, 35; Coxe, *op. cit.* (note 87), 120. Waterhouse had read Coxe's book: he quoted it in *Prospect Part II*, 32-34.

176. *Ibid.*, 16-17, 37.

177. In his letter dated Dec. 20, 1800, Waterhouse mentioned "that all the vaccine matter hitherto used in America (some received at Ipswich excepted) came from *less than two inches* of infected thread which I received from *Bath*, in *England* last June. . . ." *Independent Chronicle*, Jan. 5, 1801. But Waterhouse wrote Lettsom on Dec. 13, 1800, "I am the only person who ever succeeded in obtaining efficient matter from England. . . ." Pettigrew, *loc. cit.* (note 21), 280. Possibly this was a slip of the pen.

178. *Prospect Part II*, 38-39. Waterhouse did, however, refer to some of the tests in his newspaper articles.

179. *Prospect Part II*, 48, 51. Jackson had been Waterhouse's pupil only insofar as he had attended the medical lectures at Harvard before he went abroad. His preceptor was Dr. Edward A. Holyoke of Salem. Waterhouse did not mention the fact, well known in Boston, that Jackson had studied under Woodville.

180. Pettigrew, *op. cit.* (note 2), III, 211-212; Baron, *op. cit.*, I, 439-443. See also, Waterhouse to Ring, Aug. 6, 1801, abstracted in Ring, *op. cit.*, II, 886-889. The letter from Jenner (dated Mar. 4, 1801) to which Waterhouse referred in the reply quoted by Baron, was published in *Prospect Part II*, 110-116. From this letter Waterhouse really first learned of the proper time, according to Jenner, for taking vaccine.

181. *Prospect Part II*, 14-16, 26-27, 109-116.

182. *Ibid.*, 7.

183. *Independent Chronicle*, Jan. 5, 1801, reprinted from *Columbian Centinel*, Dec. 27, 1800. See Waterhouse, *Prospect* (Part I), 26-27. There was a similar warning in the extract of a letter from Waterhouse to a physician in the country, *Mass. Mercury*, Oct. 21, 1800, but Waterhouse did not refer to this publication in *Prospect Part II*. Waterhouse's only indication in *Prospect* (Part I) as to when he obtained the vaccine from his childrens' and servants' arms was a remark (p. 21) that he took it from "a full maturated pustule" on his three-year-old. With a typical take, this occurs about the twelfth day.

184. In the *Columbian Centinel*, June 27, 1801, Waterhouse stated that the previous year's spurious cases arose "from taking the *matter* at too late a period." See also, *ibid.*, Aug. 12, 1801. Not until the issue of Oct. 7, 1801, did he give (in a quotation from a letter from Jenner) a specific statement of the "golden rule" of vaccination: never to take the virus after the formation of the efflorescence.

185. Waterhouse was still taking vaccine as late as the eleventh day early in April, 1801. Letter to Rand, Apr. 5, 1801, *Columbian Centinel*, July 2, 1806. Some practitioners, to be sure, did take matter from suppurating ulcers, but many did not.

186. Reverend Mr. Story (Dr. Story's brother) to Waterhouse, May 7, 1801, Waterhouse, *Prospect Part II*, 12.

187. *Ibid.*, 10.
188. *Columbian Centinel*, Nov. 19, 1800.
189. *Independent Chronicle*, Jan. 5, 1801.
190. *Columbian Centinel*, Apr. 1, 1801; letter to Rand, Apr. 5, 1801, in *ibid.*, July 2, 1806.
191. *Ibid.*, July 12, 19, Aug. 6, 1806.
192. *Ibid.*, July 19, 1806.
193. Waterhouse's first such warning in the *Columbian Centinel* was actually printed Nov. 19, 1800.
194. Note the false statement that this scheme was devised *after* others were disseminating spurious vaccine.
195. *Columbian Centinel*, Dec. 12, 1807. Waterhouse also reported in this letter that he had again variolated four of his children more than seven years after their original vaccination to demonstrate its lasting efficacy. He claimed that he had from the beginning given vaccine freely to the physicians of Boston—a demonstrable falsehood. And he added opprobrious personal references to John C. Howard, which led to another newspaper squabble, but a brief one, since the editor could not perceive "the smallest use in the prolongation of the controversy. Our readers are heartily tired of it." *Ibid.*, Dec. 16, 23, 30, 1807; Jan. 2, 1808.
196. *New-England Palladium & Commercial Advertiser*, Feb. 10, 1824. The committee favored granting Waterhouse a township in Maine, but the resolution was rejected. *Columbian Centinel*, Mar. 3, 1810. A MS. note (in Waterhouse's hand?) on page 39 of the Yale Medical Library's copy of his *Information Respecting the Origin, Progress, and Efficacy of the Kine Pock Inoculation* . . . (Cambridge, 1810) charges the Essex Junto with engineering this defeat.
197. It is interesting to note that on Dec. 13, 1800, Waterhouse wrote Lettsom, "You already know, perhaps, that I introduced that distemper [cowpox] here, and led the way in its inoculation, and that very much to my advantage. . . ." Pettigrew, *loc. cit.* (note 21), 279. According to W. B. McDaniel, 2d, Waterhouse's MS. notes on John Hunter's lectures indicate that he "had a just regard for his guineas and his opportunities. . . ." "Benjamin Waterhouse's Manuscript Notes on the Lectures of John Hunter, 1777–78," *Journal of the History of Medicine and Allied Sciences*, IX (1954), 108-110.

INDEX

www.ingramcontent.com/pod-product-compliance
Lightning Source LLC
LaVergne TN
LVHW011817200926
848484LV00005B/1226